7 MINUTES TO FIT

50 ANYTIME, ANYWHERE INTERVAL WORKOUTS

Brett Klika

CHRONICLE BOOKS

SAN FRANCISCO

Text copyright © 2015 by Brett Klika.

Library of Congress Cataloging-in-Publication Data:

Klika, Brett.
  Seven minutes to fit : 50 anytime, anywhere interval workouts / Brett Klika.
    pages cm
    ISBN 978-1-4521-3847-3 — ISBN 1-4521-3847-8 1. Exercise. 2. Physical fitness. I. Title.
  GV481.K536 2015
  613.7'1—dc23

                              2014014180

Manufactured in China

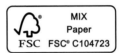

Design and illustrations by Walter C Baumann

The information, techniques, and exercises in this book are solely those of Brett Klika, a certified strength and conditioning specialist and personal trainer, who is not acting in the capacity of a doctor. The information presented in this book should not be construed as medical advice and is not meant to replace treatment by licensed health professionals. Please consult your doctor or professional health-care advisor to determine your body's needs and limitations. The writer and publisher hereby disclaim any liability from injuries resulting from following any recommendation in this book.

10 9 8 7 6 5 4 3 2 1

Chronicle Books LLC
680 Second Street
San Francisco, California 94107
www.chroniclebooks.com

DEDICATION

This book is dedicated to all of those who have helped me on my mission to bring health to the masses.

CONTENTS

Have a Few Minutes?

Let's Get Fit

IN MY WORK AS A PERSONAL TRAINER, author, and motivational speaker, I have helped tens of thousands of people from all over the world improve their health by making exercise a part of their lives. I've shown them how to enjoy exercise in boardrooms and living rooms, football fields and cornfields, sunny beaches and snowy mountaintops, trains, airplanes, and everything in between. By demonstrating how anyone can make strategic use of simple execises, I've helped everyone from Olympic athletes to overweight children transform their lives through movement.

According to the Centers for Disease Control and Prevention (CDC), regular exercise is one of the most significant things you can do for your health. Frequent exercisers experience a decreased likelihood of heart disease, certain types of cancer, type 2 diabetes, depression, sleep irregularity, osteoporosis, neurological dysfunction, and a host of other health problems.

While it's widely accepted that physical activity from daily exercise can improve health, I still encounter resistance from the time-strapped, energy-deprived masses who struggle to find the minutes or motivation to "get to the gym." The good news for all is that exercise need not be confined to the gyms, tracks, and studios of the world. A beneficial workout requires no special equipment, costs nothing, and is accessible to anyone with a floor and a chair.

Even better news from researchers in the field of health and human performance is that we don't need to exercise for long periods of time to achieve the health, fitness, and body we strive for. In as little as a few seconds, exercise has been shown to improve mood and mental focus. In just a few minutes, we can improve markers of fitness (heart health, insulin sensitivity, and metabolic function) and drastically increase circulating levels of "feel-good" neurotransmitters. In less than thirty minutes of high-intensity exercise, we can positively impact our metabolism for up to seventy-two hours, decrease our likelihood of early death, increase the number of fat-burning enzymes in our muscle, improve our glucose metabolism, and decrease body fat.

All this in just a few minutes out of your day! That time before the kids wake up or after they go to bed, the thirty minutes you have at lunch, the twenty-minute study break—all of these situations could become opportunities to improve your health and energy.

7 Minutes to Fit will help you break down the barriers that prevent most people from exercising: the need for more minutes, money, or motivation to go to the gym. These pages will show you that with the right kind of approach and the best piece of exercise equipment ever created—your body—you can get stronger, become more fit, and burn body fat in the few minutes your busy life affords you. You're holding the blueprint in your hands!

High-Intensity Interval Training: More Results, Less Time

Strategic, high-intensity workouts are often cited in the research on efficient exercise. This type of regimen, known as "high-intensity interval training," is currently being used by millions of people around the world to get results from exercise in a short amount of time.

Standard interval training—originally used to improve the performance of track athletes—raises your heart rate for a period of time, followed by a period of time when your heart rate decreases, or "recovers." This is repeated a number of times. For example, you could perform an exercise for one minute, then rest for one minute, and then repeat that process ten times.

In *high-intensity* interval training, you significantly elevate your heart rate, usually to about 90 percent of your maximum, for a short period of time. Recovery time is usually either at full rest or at an intensity at or below about 70 percent of your maximum heart rate. Interval training and high-intensity interval training programs are alternatives to long-duration, low-intensity aerobic training, which has long been embraced by the fitness crowd.

Various studies comparing low-intensity, long-duration work to high-intensity interval training have demonstrated that the latter may be more efficient in burning fat and improving fitness. Scientists in Australia recently found that high-intensity interval training for sixty minutes per week resulted in the same amount of fat loss as seven hours of low-intensity work. In other words, better results in far less time!

I saw the universal appeal for this more efficient approach to exercise when I coauthored a review on the benefits of short-duration, high-intensity interval training for the American College of Sports Medicine. The *New York Times* published the review and coined it "The Scientific 7-Minute Workout." The article quickly went viral, and now a search for "7-minute workout" yields nearly 100 million results on Google.

How to Use This Book *7 Minutes to Fit* presents fifty effective and targeted interval workouts that range from focusing on a single area of the body to providing an invigorating calorie-burning full-body challenge. I have drawn from more than fifteen years of personal experience creating customized workouts to present exercises that work for people at all skill levels and focus on different parts of the body. To get started, I have created a glossary of forty-one exercises you can do with just your body weight and a chair. Each exercise is carefully described and includes an illustration to show exactly how you should perform the movement. While you might recognize some of these movements from your days in phys ed, sports practice, or exercise class, you may not know that these are among the most powerful exercises for raising your heart rate and changing your body. When used in the right combinations with strategic intensity, these exercises can yield impressive results. As you begin, make sure to read and follow the glossary descriptions and perform each movement with the correct technique, so that your exercise is safe and effective.

Once you've mastered the basic movements, it's time to dive into the fifty high-intensity interval workouts. These bodyweight workouts are organized so you can choose to work your entire body or target a specific area, such as your arms, legs, or abs. Even for these more targeted workouts, nearly every muscle is involved to some degree, in order to create a balanced body. This not only provides a unique challenge, but also prevents injuries and improves posture.

Fifty different exercise routines enable you to choose a different workout every day for nearly two months. That means every day you'll have a new strategy to maximize your health in minimal time. So much for exercise being repetitive and boring! Plus, at the end of the book, I have listed ways to vary the workouts to allow for even more exercise options. As you can see, your opportunity for variety is endless. And with no equipment necessary, you can exercise anywhere, at your own pace. Take this book with you when you're on the road, or leave it by your nightstand for a quick morning boost.

With this little book, there's nothing complicated. Just move, sweat, add variety, and repeat. The recipe for ongoing health and vitality is that simple. No equipment, no driving to the gym, and no guesswork. Just carefully designed, fun, and challenging programs that can be done anywhere. And remember: exercise is not an event; it's a lifestyle. The important thing is that your body and brain draw the connection that "movement makes me feel good, so I'm going to do it whenever I can." With that mind-set, you will be a happy, healthy exerciser for life.

Enjoy the process of health as you sweat, smile, and sustain your vitality for the rest of your life using only your body—the one piece of equipment you never leave behind. I'm honored to be part of your journey.

PART ONE

MOVEMENT GLOSSARY

In this section, you will find step-by-step instructions for all of the exercises included in the fifty high-intensity bodyweight work-outs in part two. Nearly all the included exercises require strength, coordination, and flexibility of the entire body as a unit. While some exercises focus on certain areas of the body, most require the inte-gration of the lower body, upper body, and core to be done correctly and effectively. Refer to this handy chart to know which part of the body each movement targets:

TARGETED MOVEMENTS

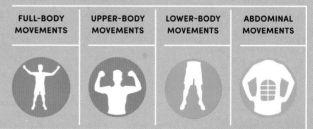

FULL-BODY MOVEMENTS	UPPER-BODY MOVEMENTS	LOWER-BODY MOVEMENTS	ABDOMINAL MOVEMENTS

These exercises were strategically selected because they are extremely effective. Nearly all of them increase the heart rate while improving strength and flexibility. If you find that any particular exercise is painful or too advanced for you, simply select another exercise for that body part. Each exercise notes the specific body part it targets, so you can swap them out if needed. If Lateral Lunges are too difficult, choose another lower-body exercise that works better for you, such as Reverse Lunges. Practice the exercises at your own pace, but remember that when you advance to the fifty detailed workouts, you'll perform each exercise for thirty seconds with a ten-second rest.

10s AND 2s

This abdominal exercise targets the hard-to-reach lateral area of the abdomen.

1 Lie on your back with legs together, extended straight up toward the ceiling, perpendicular to the floor. Arms should be straight out to the sides of the body, forming a T position.

2 Keeping legs together and the arms out to the side, rotate legs side to side from a ten o'clock position to a two o'clock position.

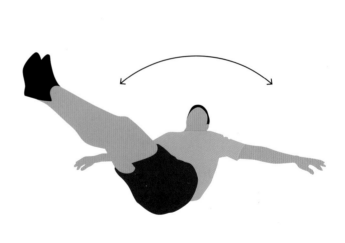

AGILITY CIRCLES

Agility Circles will increase your heart rate and provide a unique challenge.

1 Place this book on the floor and stand about 6 inches/15 cm in front of the book.

2 Begin moving your feet quickly while facing forward, moving in a clockwise circle around the book as quickly as possible.

3 Once you have completed a clockwise rotation, return in a counterclockwise direction as quickly as possible.

4 Repeat, alternating clockwise and counterclockwise motions, taking care to face forward the entire time (i.e., do not run in a circle).

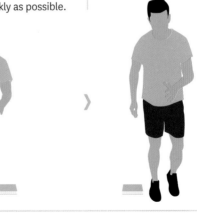

ALTERNATING SUPERMANS

Alternating Supermans develop the muscles of the back.

1 Lie facedown on the ground with arms straight out in front of the body (imagine yourself as Superman flying).

2 Keeping both arms and legs straight and the chin tucked toward the chest, raise the left arm and right leg simultaneously, holding for a brief moment at the top of the motion.

3 Return to the start position and repeat with the right arm and left leg.

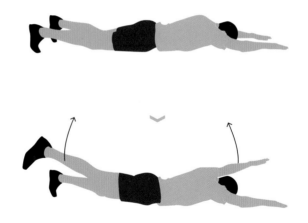

BALANCE REACHES

In addition to working your balance, this exercise focuses on hip flexibility, mobility, and strength.

1 Stand on your right leg with your right knee slightly bent.

2 Without further flexing your right knee, bend at the hip and reach forward with your left arm while straightening and raising your left leg behind you. Bend and reach until your torso and left leg are as close to parallel with the ground as possible, with the hip also remaining parallel to the ground.

3 Remain on the right leg for 30 seconds without the left foot touching the ground. Then repeat the exercise on the left leg for 30 seconds.

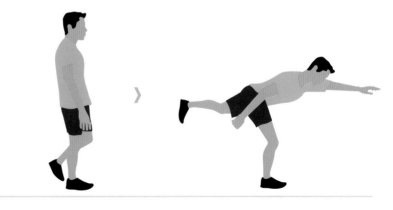

BICYCLES

Bicycles incorporate the upper, lower, and side areas of the abs.

1 Lie on your back with hands clasped behind your head to support the neck, elbows flat to the ground away from the head.

2 Bend your knees and lift the feet off the ground, bringing knees toward the chest, so that the thighs form a 90-degree angle with the torso.

3 Using this as the start position, simultaneously lift the upper torso (as if to perform a Crunch) and rotate to bring the left knee toward the right elbow.

4 Once the left knee and right elbow come as close to contact as possible, return to the start position and repeat with opposite knee/elbow in a controlled manner.

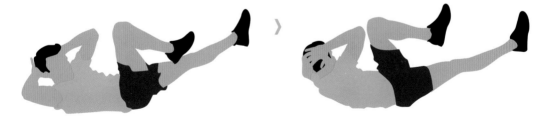

BURPEES

Burpees increase your heart rate while burning calories.

1 Begin by standing upright with arms straight up in the air.

2 Squat down and place hands on the ground outside of the feet.

3 Jump both legs back in one motion, ending in a Push-Up position (see page 37).

4 Return to a squat by hopping both knees back toward the chest, ending in the same position as in Step 2.

5 Return to the start position and repeat.

CROSS-BODY V-UPS

Cross-Body V-Ups require the hips, abs, and shoulders to work together.

1 Begin by lying flat on your back, with arms straight out to the side and legs outstretched to form a V shape on the floor.

2 Raise the upper body as if doing a Crunch. Simultaneously lift the left arm and right leg, bringing them toward each other in a cross-body motion, taking care to keep the leg and arm straight. The right arm and left leg should remain on the ground.

3 Once the left hand touches the right foot, lower the body back to the start position and repeat the motion with the opposite leg/arm.

CRUNCHES

Crunches create strong abs while minimizing stress on the neck and lower back.

1 Begin by lying with your back flat on the ground, knees bent, with the soles of your feet on the floor. Your hands are behind the head and used as support for the neck during the movement, but they should not pull the neck forward.

2 Slowly peel your spine off the ground, raising the chest toward the ceiling.

3 Once you have raised the chest as high as possible without using momentum, return to the start position and repeat.

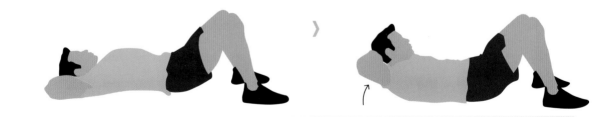

CURTSY LUNGES

This movement works the hips and gluteal muscles while increasing flexibility.

1 Begin standing upright, with legs slightly farther than shoulder-width apart.

2 Keeping the hips forward, step the left leg behind the right leg laterally. The legs will cross.

3 Once the left leg has reached as far as possible and is placed on the ground without the hips twisting, lower the left knee to the ground. This motion should be similar to a curtsy.

4 Return to the start position, alternate legs, and repeat on the other side.

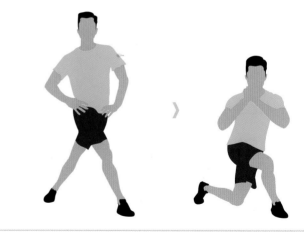

DIAGONAL LUNGES

Like Curtsy Lunges, Diagonal Lunges work the hips and gluteal muscles. The different angle for each lunge creates a different flexibility and strength requirement.

1 Begin standing upright, with legs slightly farther than shoulder-width apart.

2 Keeping the hips forward, step the left leg in front of the right leg laterally. The legs will cross.

3 Once the left leg has reached as far as possible across the body's midline and the foot is placed on the ground while the hips remain forward, lower the right knee to the ground.

4 Return to the start position, alternate legs, and repeat on the other side.

DIVE-BOMBER PUSH-UPS

This advanced Push-Up variation concentrates greater focus on the shoulder muscles.

1 Begin in a Push-Up position (see page 37).

2 Raise the hips significantly above parallel to ground, so that your butt is in the air.

3 Begin lowering the body toward the ground, keeping hips elevated, leading with the head, facing the ground.

4 As you approach the ground, begin to lower your hips and shift your weight forward, so that your shoulders move over your hands.

5 Raise your head and chest until your arms are straight, while keeping your hips as close as possible to the ground.

6 Once your arms are straight, with chest and head up, reverse the motion by shifting your weight so your shoulders move back behind the hands while you raise your hips to the starting position above, parallel. Then repeat.

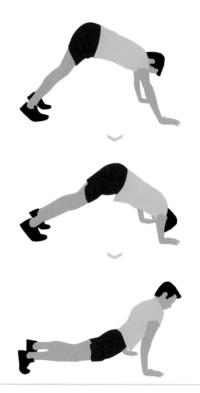

DOUBLE CRUNCHES

This advanced version of standard Crunches challenges the lower and upper abdominals.

1 Begin with the setup for a Crunch (see page 18).

2 Begin the Crunch motion and simultaneously lift your feet off the ground, bringing your bent knees toward your chest.

3 Once the knees and the chest come as close together as possible, at a point above the waistline, return to the start position and repeat.

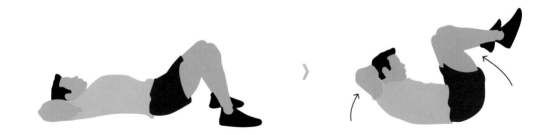

HELLO DOLLIES

This exercise strengthens the hips and abs.

1 Lie on your back with hands clasped behind head, elbows away from head.

2 Raise both legs together until they are perpendicular to the ground.

3 Begin peeling the spine off the ground, raising the chest toward the ceiling.

4 As you lift the chest toward the ceiling, open your legs as far apart as possible.

5 Keeping the abs flexed and still pushing the chest toward the ceiling, bring the legs back together.

6 Once the legs are together, lower your upper body to the start position and repeat.

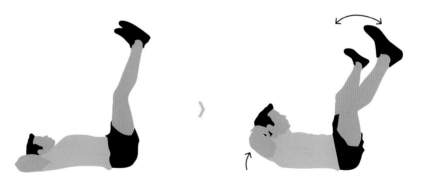

HIGHTAIL PUSH-UPS

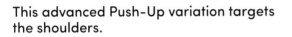

This advanced Push-Up variation targets the shoulders.

1 Start in a Dive-Bomber Push-Up position (see page 21).

2 Begin lowering your body toward the ground, keeping hips elevated, leading with the head, facing the ground.

3 Keep hips elevated as high as possible as you bring your forehead toward the ground.

4 Once you have gotten your forehead as close to the ground as possible, push up to return to the start position, with the hips elevated high in the air, and repeat.

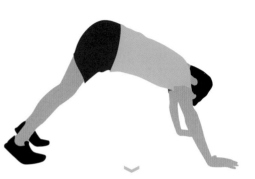

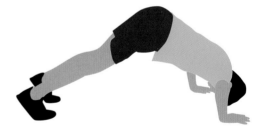

JUMP LUNGES

This advanced Lunge variation improves strength and muscle tone in the legs while increasing the heart rate.

1 Begin by stepping your left foot forward and doing a Lunge (see page 29).

2 Once you have lowered yourself as much as you can, raise your center as quickly as possible. At the top of the movement, leave the ground in a jump.

3 While both feet are off the ground, alternate them, so you land with the right foot forward.

4 Repeat the lunge, jump, and switch motion with the right foot forward.

JUMP SQUATS

This advanced Squat variation improves strength and muscle tone in the legs while increasing the heart rate.

1 Begin by doing a Squat (see page 44).

2 Once you have lowered yourself as much as possible, jump up as high as possible.

3 Land from the jump in a Squat position, with legs bent. Then repeat.

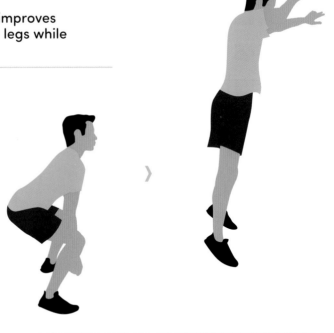

JUMPING JACKS

Jumping Jacks raise your heart rate quickly, increasing your ability to burn fat.

1 Begin standing upright with feet together, arms hanging straight down on either side.

2 Hop the legs apart while simultaneously bringing the arms up laterally from the body, so that the palms touch above the head when the feet land outside of shoulder width.

3 Rapidly return to the starting position by hopping the legs back together and returning the arms straight down to the side.

4 Repeat in a rhythmic manner.

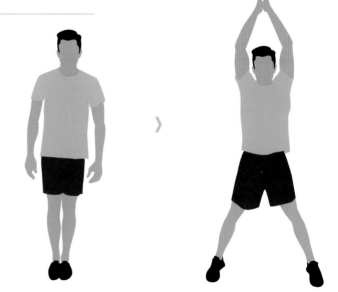

LATERAL LUNGES

Lateral Lunges improve flexibility and strengthen inner and outer thighs.

1 Begin by standing upright, with feet farther than shoulder-width apart.

2 Bend the left knee to shift the hips laterally to the left, keeping the torso upright and the right leg straight.

3 As the left knee bends, the hips lower until they reach the lowest point possible, with the gluteals directly over the left heel.

4 Return to the start position, alternate legs, and repeat on the other side.

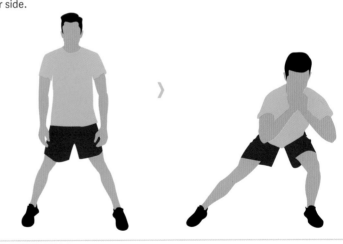

LUNGES

Lunges increase lower-body strength and flexibility while improving muscle tone.

1 Begin by standing upright with feet together.

2 Step forward with the left foot as far as possible.

3 When the foot is placed on the ground, begin bending both knees, lowering your center toward the ground. The left knee bends, but does not move forward over the toes. Continue until the right knee nearly touches the ground.

4 Once you have lowered yourself as much as possible, return to standing position.

5 Repeat with the right foot stepping forward.

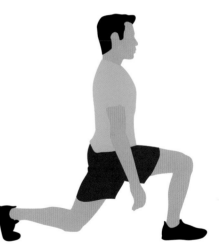

MOUNTAIN CLIMBERS

Mountain Climbers improve core strength while increasing the heart rate.

1 Begin in a Push-Up position (see page 37).

2 Rapidly bring the right knee up to the chest while maintaining the Push-Up position.

3 When the right knee is as close to the chest as possible, begin extending your leg while simultaneously bringing the other knee to your chest.

4 Rapidly alternate this motion.

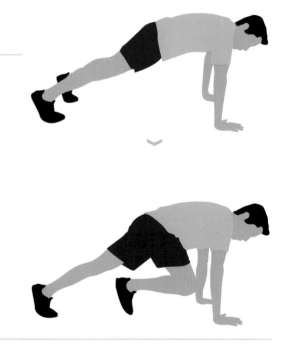

PLANK

Plank improves core strength and posture without placing extra stress on the lower back.

1 Begin by lying on your stomach on the floor, propping up your upper body on your elbows and forearms.

2 Lift the hips and straighten the legs, so that only your elbows, forearms, and toes are in contact with the ground. Spine remains straight and hips remain parallel to the ground.

3 Maintain this position for the duration of the exercise, with hips parallel to the ground, and spine and legs straight.

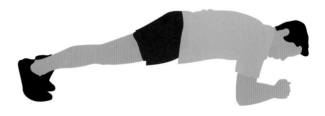

PLANK TO PUSH-UP

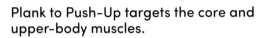

Plank to Push-Up targets the core and upper-body muscles.

1 Set up in a Plank position (see page 31).

2 Slightly shift your weight to the left forearm/elbow while placing the palm of the right hand on the ground.

3 Push the palm of the right hand into the ground and straighten the right elbow, as if doing a Push-Up.

4 Once the right elbow begins to straighten, repeat on the left side, ending in a Push-Up position.

5 Once you reach a Push-Up position, return to the start position by bending the right elbow, then the left. Repeat the movement beginning with the weight on the right forearm/elbow and straightening the left arm.

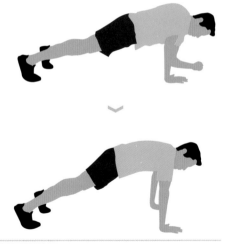

PRIMAL STEP-UPS

Primal Step-Ups improve lower-body flexibility and strength.

1 Perform a Reverse Lunge (see page 39) with the right leg stepping back.

2 As your knee moves toward the ground, reach toward the ground with both hands, ending with the left hand as close as possible to the inside of the left foot.

3 Once the hand contacts the ground, continue bending the left knee and attempt to lower the chest toward the ground in a Push-Up motion.

4 During this motion, the heel of the left foot stays in contact with the ground and the right leg remains as straight as possible as it extends behind the body.

5 Once you've lowered your chest as far as possible, keeping the heel of the left foot on the ground, return to the start position in one motion by pushing with both arms while simultaneously bringing the right leg back to meet the left leg in a standing position.

6 Alternate and repeat on the other side.

PRISONERS

Prisoners improve your upper-back strength and posture.

1 Begin lying facedown on the ground with the hands clasped behind the head.

2 Keeping your head tucked toward the chest (as if you were holding a tennis ball under your chin), raise the chest off the ground, keeping the legs and feet in contact with the ground.

3 Return to the start position and repeat.

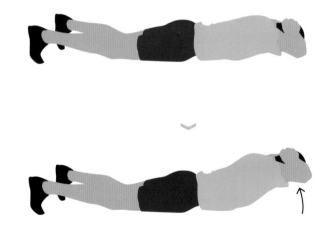

PUSH-UP AND ROTATE

This advanced Push-Up variation strengthens the entire upper body and core.

1 Begin by doing a Push-Up (see page 37).

2 At the top of the motion (once the arms are straight), lift the right hand and leg off the ground and rotate, so that your body is perpendicular to the ground, with your weight being supported by the left hand and foot. The right arm and leg remain straight as you lift them off the ground. The spine remains straight as well.

3 Reach your right arm and leg toward the ceiling, pause for a moment, then return to the starting position.

4 Repeat the entire Push-Up movement, lifting the left arm and leg.

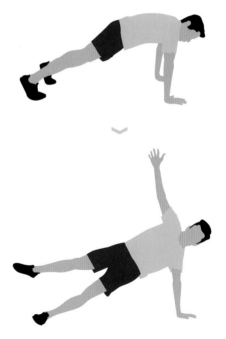

PUSH-UP SPIDERS

Push-Up Spiders combine upper-body and core strength.

1 Begin by doing a Push-Up (see page 37).

2 At the top of the motion (once the arms are straight), bring the right hand and left foot off the ground.

3 Bend the left leg to bring the knee toward the chest while simultaneously reaching to the left foot with the right hand, under the body. Keep hips parallel to the ground.

4 Once the right hand and left foot touch in a controlled manner, return to the starting position and repeat the movement with your right knee and left hand.

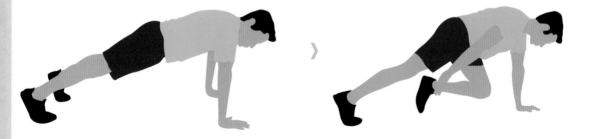

PUSH-UPS

Push-Ups increase chest, shoulder, triceps, and core strength.

1 Begin in a Push-Up position, with hands and feet on the floor, knees off the ground, back flat, legs straight, and shoulders directly over the hands.

2 Lower your chest toward the ground in a slow, controlled fashion.

3 Once you have lowered yourself as much as possible, use your upper-body and core strength to return to the starting position in Step 1. Then repeat.

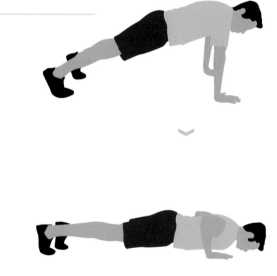

REVERSE LUNGE AND ROTATE

The Reverse Lunge and Rotate combines core and lower-body strength.

1 Begin by standing upright, feet at shoulder width or slightly wider, arms straight out in front of the body with hands clasped.

2 Perform a Reverse Lunge (see page 39) with the right leg, keeping the arms outstretched to the front, hands clasped.

3 As the right knee bends to approach the ground, simultaneously rotate the torso toward the left knee, keeping the arms outstretched and the upper body upright.

4 Return to the start position after the right knee touches the ground and repeat the motion beginning with the left leg.

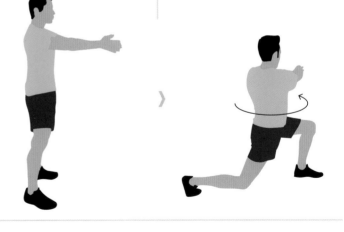

REVERSE LUNGES

Reverse Lunges improve strength, flexibility, and muscle tone of the lower body.

1 Begin by standing upright with feet together.

2 Step back with the right leg as far as possible.

3 Once the right foot contacts the ground at a point behind the body, lower the right knee to the ground, keeping the upper body upright and the heel of the front foot on the ground.

4 When the right knee touches the ground, return to the start position and repeat on the left side.

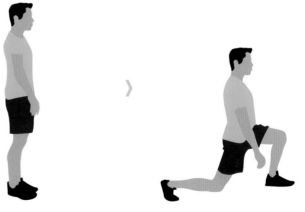

SHADOW BOXING

Shadow Boxing requires upper- and lower-body agility and coordination.

1 Begin by standing with one foot in front of the other, about shoulder-width apart, knees bent, weight on the balls of the feet.

2 Create fists with both hands and bring them in front of the face, in a boxer's position, with the elbows bent.

3 Begin alternating punches with the right and left hands while you move your feet forward, back, and side to side in a random fashion.

4 Mix the cadence and types of punches. For example, do two left-hand punches followed by a right-hand, then switch. Every five to ten punches, add a squat to dodge an imaginary opponent's punch. Attempt to execute about thirty punches in thirty seconds.

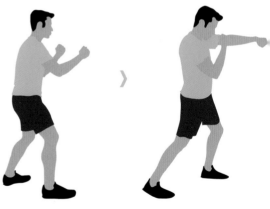

SIDE PLANK

Side Plank helps develop the strength of the muscles on the lateral areas of the body.

1 Begin by lying on your right side, propping up the upper body with the right elbow and forearm.

2 Lift the right hip off the ground, resulting in your weight being supported by the right elbow/forearm and side of the right foot. Spine remains straight, shoulder blades remain retracted, and upper body is perpendicular to the floor.

3 Maintain this position for the duration of the exercise.

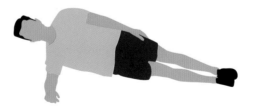

SKATER PLYOS

Skater Plyos help strengthen the gluteals and other muscles of the outer thigh.

1 Begin by balancing on the left leg with the knee slightly bent.

2 Push off laterally with the left leg, landing on the right foot.

3 Achieve balance on the right leg by slightly bending the right knee.

4 Once you achieve balance, push off with the right leg laterally, landing on the left foot.

5 Repeat in a speed-skating motion.

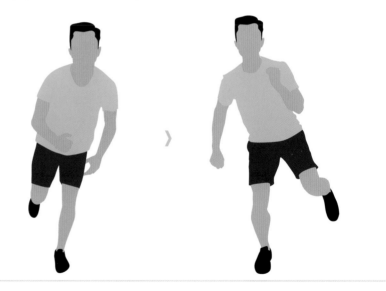

SPORTS SPRINTS

Sports Sprints help increase the heart rate and strengthen running muscles.

1 Stand upright with arms bent at 90 degrees.

2 When time starts, begin running in place. Attempt to bring each ankle to the height of the opposite knee while running as quickly as possible in place.

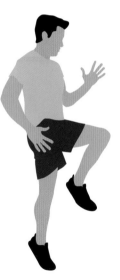

SQUATS

Squats increase flexibility, strength, and muscle tone of the gluteals and quads.

1 Begin standing with feet slightly farther than shoulder-width apart.

2 Shift the hips backward, as if trying to shut a car door with your butt.

3 Simultaneously begin bending the knees, lowering your center toward the ground. Your spine remains straight and parallel with your shins.

4 Lower yourself as much as possible, keeping spine parallel to shins, feet entirely on the floor, and knees behind toes.

5 Once you have lowered yourself as much as you can, stand up to return to the start position. Then repeat.

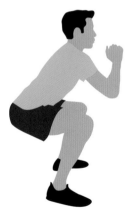

STEP-UP SQUATS

Step-Up Squats improve lower-body strength and flexibility.

1 Beginning in a Push-Up position (see page 37), bend the left knee to bring the left foot as close to the outside of the left hand as possible. Then do the same with the right foot.

2 Once both feet are in place near the hands, with the heels on the ground, reach the left hand straight up as high as possible, followed by the right hand, so that both hands are reaching upward. As you reach, chest and head should remain upright, heels remain on the ground, and the arms remain straight.

3 Maintaining this position with the chest, arms, and head, move to a standing position.

4 Bring arms back down and return to the bottom of the Squat position, placing both hands on the ground.

5 Step the left, then the right foot back to the start position. Then repeat, leading with the other foot.

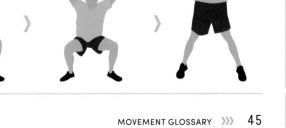

SURFERS

Surfers improve upper- and lower-body strength and coordination.

1 Begin by lying facedown on the ground, with palms on the ground, as if getting ready to do a Push-Up.

2 Using the upper body, lower body, and trunk, jump to your feet as quickly as possible, landing in a Squat position, with one leg in front of the other, body slightly sideways, as if riding a surfboard.

3 Return to a facedown position and repeat with the other leg landing forward.

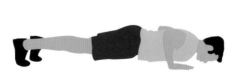

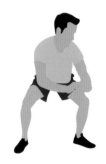

SWIMMERS

Swimmers help strengthen the muscles of the upper back and shoulders.

1 Begin in the Alternating Supermans position (see page 13) with arms and hands outstretched in front of the body.

2 Lift the hands and arms off the ground, while keeping the feet in contact with the ground, and perform a front crawl swimming motion without allowing the hands and arms to touch the ground.

3 During the movement, keep the head tucked as if you were holding a tennis ball between your chin and neck.

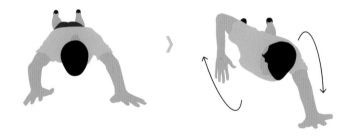

TOE TOUCHES

Toe Touches improve the strength of the upper-abdominal region.

1 Lie on your back with legs outstretched and arms raised perpendicular to the ground.

2 Lift both legs until they are perpendicular to the ground.

3 Keeping the legs perpendicular to the ground and the arms straight, reach your hands toward your toes.

4 Once your hands come as close as possible to your toes, return your upper back to the floor while keeping your legs straight up and perpendicular to the ground and repeat.

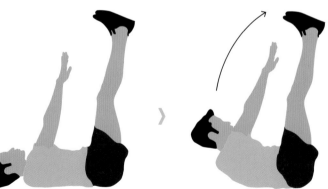

TRICEPS DIP AND REACH

This advanced version of the Triceps Dip increases the challenge to the triceps muscles.

1 Perform a Triceps Dip exercise (see page 50).

2 Once you reach the top of the motion (elbows straight), remove your right hand from the chair and reach toward the ceiling, so that your entire body weight is on your left hand. Your upper body will twist as you reach.

3 Return to the start position and repeat on the other side.

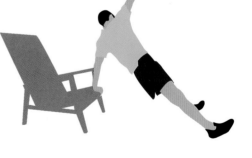

TRICEPS DIPS

Triceps Dips develop the triceps muscles found on the back of the upper arms.

1 Start by sitting on the edge of a stable chair. Place the palms of the hands on the corners of the chair, fingers facing forward.

2 Walk your legs out, so you are no longer resting on the edge of the chair.

3 Straighten the legs, so your weight is supported by the hands and heels.

4 Lower your body by bending the elbows.

5 Once you have lowered your body as much as possible, push your body back up to the start position, with your hands and heels supporting your weight. Then repeat.

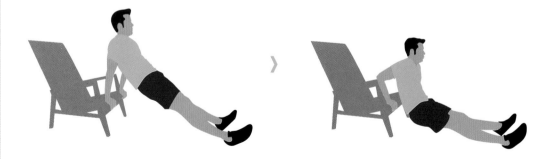

WORM WALKOUTS

Worm Walkouts require strength and coordination of upper- and lower-body muscles.

1 Begin by standing upright, with feet shoulder-width apart.

2 Perform a Squat (see page 44) and place hands on the ground inside of the feet at the bottom of the motion.

3 Once the hands make contact with the ground, walk them out in front of the feet as far as possible, preferably to a point where your hands are well out in front of your body, both legs are straight, and the torso is parallel to the ground.

4 Once the hands are out as far as possible, bend the knees and walk the hands back to the bottom of the Squat position, then return to the start position and repeat.

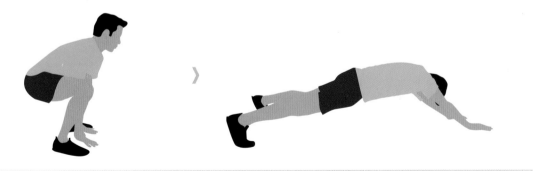

PART TWO

FIFTY BODYWEIGHT WORKOUTS YOU CAN DO ANYWHERE

Now that you've had a chance to practice all the exercises, it's time to put them to use with the fifty unique workouts in this book. As you will see, the workouts are divided into body part focuses: Full-Body Workouts, Upper-Body Workouts, Lower-Body Workouts, and Abdominal Workouts.

Workouts have a majority of their exercises focusing on a specific area of the body, but every workout includes at least one exercise for each body part. This is to ensure that regardless of the workouts you choose to perform, you are balancing all the muscles in your body.

Everyone has different exercise preferences, as well as strengths and weaknesses in different muscles of the body. It is recommended that you perform at least one of each of the full-body, upper-body, and lower-body workouts per week. Abdominal exercises are an inherent part of every workout, so it is not necessary to perform a specific abdominal workout every week.

Performing the Workouts

ALL THE INCLUDED WORKOUTS ARE designed to have you perform each movement for thirty seconds, to elevate your heart rate to the high-intensity range, with ten seconds of rest in between movements. This ten-second rest period allows just enough time for a short recovery. A recovery period enables you to achieve a high level of intensity during the intervals. Without a rest between these high-intensity bouts, significant fatigue would set in and you would have to decrease the intensity in order to finish the workout. If the rest period is too long, your body doesn't experience enough stress to force a change.

To repeat the workout multiple times, allow thirty seconds between each round (also known as a circuit). Never feel as if you have to rush through exercises. Doing it right is what will make the difference in your health. Also, multiple circuits in a workout do not have to merely be repetitions of the same workout. For example, you could perform a circuit of an upper-body workout, follow with a full-body workout, and finish with an abdominal circuit to get three total circuits in twenty minutes. With exercise combinations, you have nearly unending options for variety.

The workouts are designed to be done without equipment. However, prior to beginning a workout you should have the following:

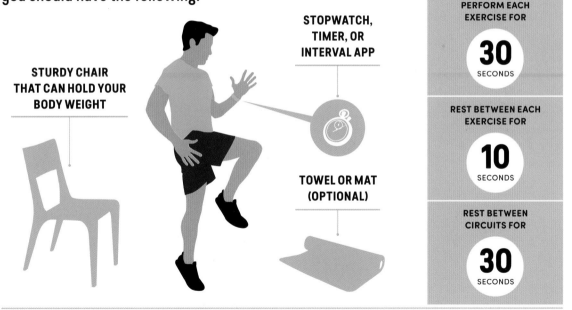

STURDY CHAIR THAT CAN HOLD YOUR BODY WEIGHT

STOPWATCH, TIMER, OR INTERVAL APP

TOWEL OR MAT (OPTIONAL)

To complete the workout:

PERFORM EACH EXERCISE FOR

30 SECONDS

REST BETWEEN EACH EXERCISE FOR

10 SECONDS

REST BETWEEN CIRCUITS FOR

30 SECONDS

Take Your Time These programs were designed with you, the busy, time-strapped adult, in mind. Sometimes you have twenty minutes to dedicate to exercise, while at other times you may barely have five. That's why I've included three options, depending on the amount of time you have to exercise. In all of these circuits, you'll keep your heart rate elevated by moving from one exercise to the next, resting only the allotted ten seconds between exercises. Here are the benefits you'll get from each circuit round:

ONE CIRCUIT	UNDER SEVEN MINUTES	TWO CIRCUITS	UNDER FIFTEEN MINUTES	THREE CIRCUITS	ABOUT TWENTY MINUTES
Boost energy, clear "brain fog," feel great.		Improve heart, lung, and brain health; increase overall fitness.		Burn fat, shape the body, lose weight, significantly improve health and well-being.	
Quite often, just getting started with a program is the toughest part, so beginning with a quick five-, six-, or seven-minute workout may be the way to go. Even this short stint of exercise will give you an energy boost. You'll feel great, and, who knows, it may lead to longer workouts in the future.		Research has shown that in as little as about fifteen minutes, you can improve your heart, lungs, and brain, in addition to significantly increasing your feel-good hormones.		Twenty minutes of carefully designed, targeted exercise can effect dramatic health, energy, and body improvements.	

To get the maximum health and fitness benefits, I recommend completing three circuits whenever possible. When you first start exercising, you may not be able to achieve that—that's completely normal—and you may need to work your way up to three circuits. It will give you something to strive for. Performing these workouts three to four days per week, in addition to any other active hobbies you have, is also ideal. While these are the guidelines I recommend, never forget that merely getting *some* movement on a daily basis will change your life for the better. If you miss a day, or can only exercise for a few minutes on any given day, that's OK.

It's time to get started with these workouts you can perform anywhere to improve your health, your body, and your life!

A Safe Intensity for You I create fitness programs for people at all different fitness levels because no single program is right for everyone. It's important to meet with your doctor prior to starting any fitness program, particularly a program that includes high-intensity training like this one. Once you've received a clean bill of health, be sure to tailor your exercise program to determine the safest, most effective intensity for your training. The intensity of exercise is what ultimately determines its safety, effectiveness, and efficiency. Monitoring your heart rate and how you feel during exercise are the most common ways to measure exercise intensity. Talk to your doctor about determining the safest, most effective exercise heart rate for you. And always pay attention to how you feel during your workouts. Exercising at intensities that make you sick, dizzy, or otherwise impaired can have a serious negative effect on your health. Regardless of the hype, it actually does more harm than good and is not recommended.

FULL-BODY WORKOUTS
MAXIMUM CALORIE BURN

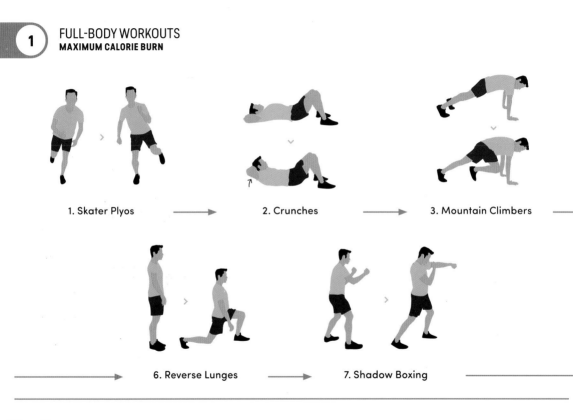

1. Skater Plyos $\longrightarrow$ 2. Crunches $\longrightarrow$ 3. Mountain Climbers $\longrightarrow$

$\longrightarrow$ 6. Reverse Lunges $\longrightarrow$ 7. Shadow Boxing $\longrightarrow$

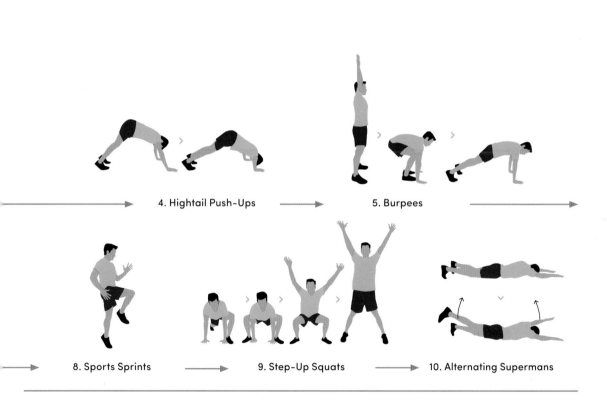

4. Hightail Push-Ups

5. Burpees

8. Sports Sprints

9. Step-Up Squats

10. Alternating Supermans

2

FULL-BODY WORKOUTS
MAXIMUM CALORIE BURN

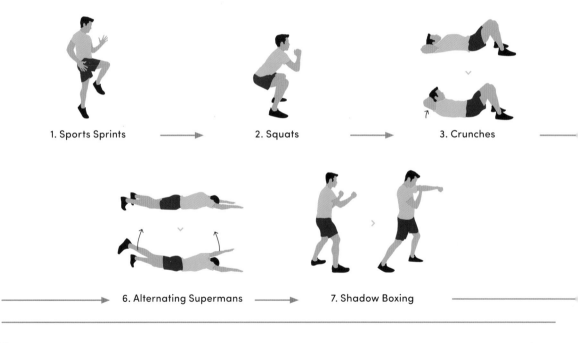

1. Sports Sprints → 2. Squats → 3. Crunches →

6. Alternating Supermans → 7. Shadow Boxing

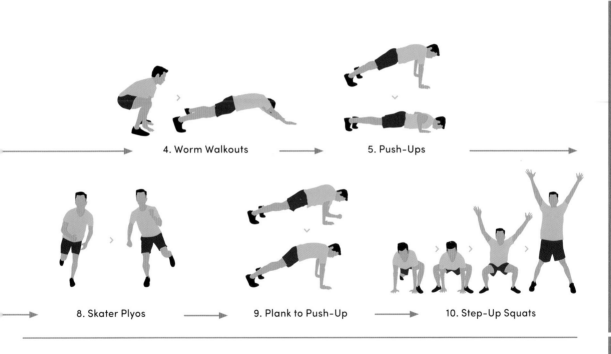

4. Worm Walkouts

5. Push-Ups

8. Skater Plyos

9. Plank to Push-Up

10. Step-Up Squats

FULL-BODY WORKOUTS
MAXIMUM CALORIE BURN

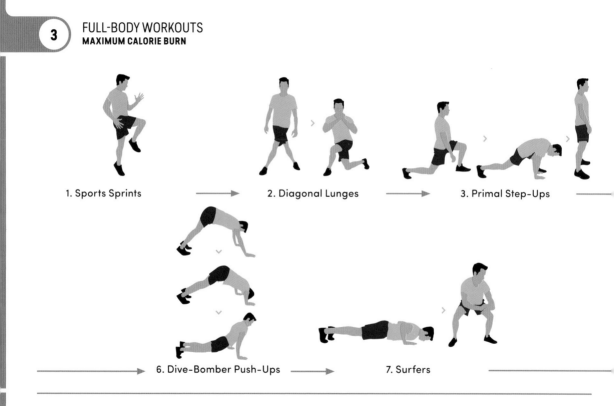

1. Sports Sprints

2. Diagonal Lunges

3. Primal Step-Ups

6. Dive-Bomber Push-Ups

7. Surfers

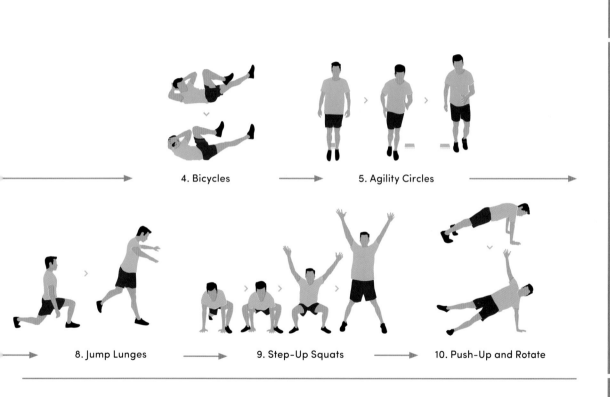

4. Bicycles

5. Agility Circles

8. Jump Lunges

9. Step-Up Squats

10. Push-Up and Rotate

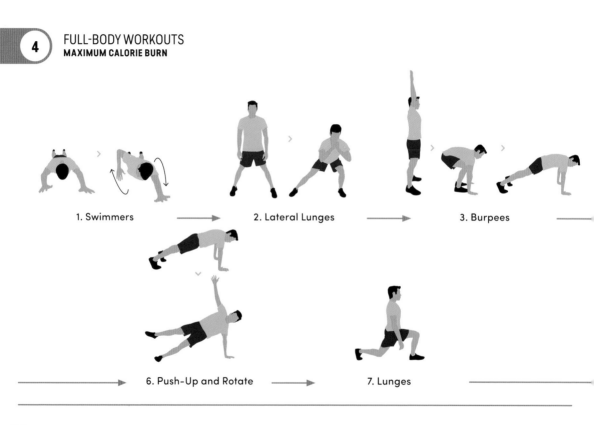

1. Swimmers → 2. Lateral Lunges → 3. Burpees →

→ 6. Push-Up and Rotate → 7. Lunges →

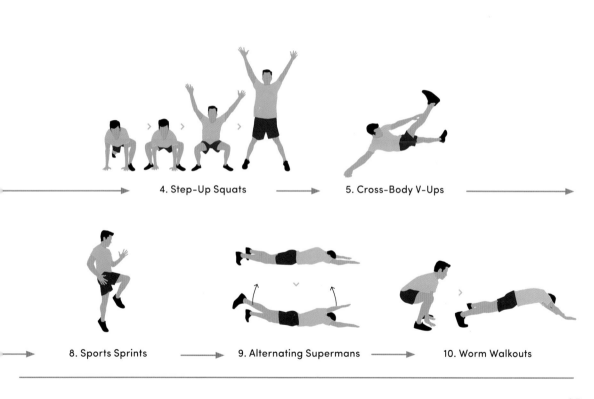

4. Step-Up Squats

5. Cross-Body V-Ups

8. Sports Sprints

9. Alternating Supermans

10. Worm Walkouts

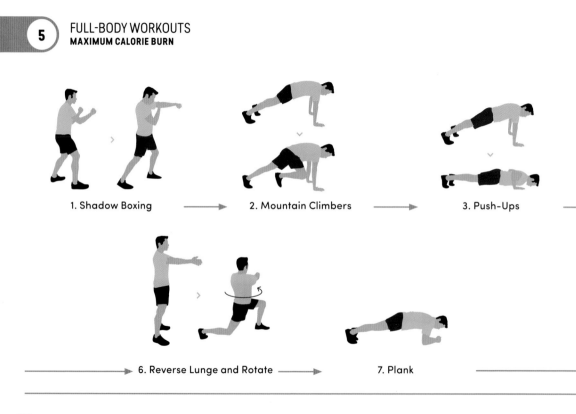

1. Shadow Boxing ⟶ 2. Mountain Climbers ⟶ 3. Push-Ups ⟶

⟶ 6. Reverse Lunge and Rotate ⟶ 7. Plank

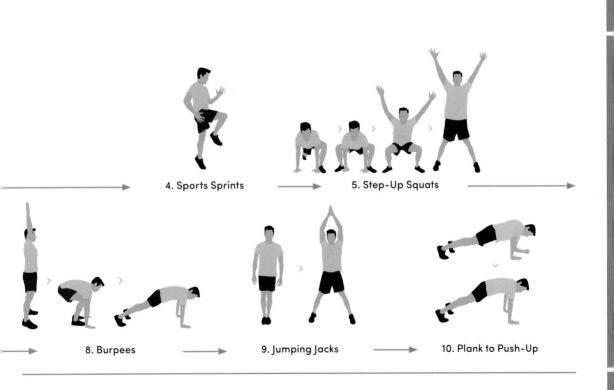

4. Sports Sprints

5. Step-Up Squats

8. Burpees

9. Jumping Jacks

10. Plank to Push-Up

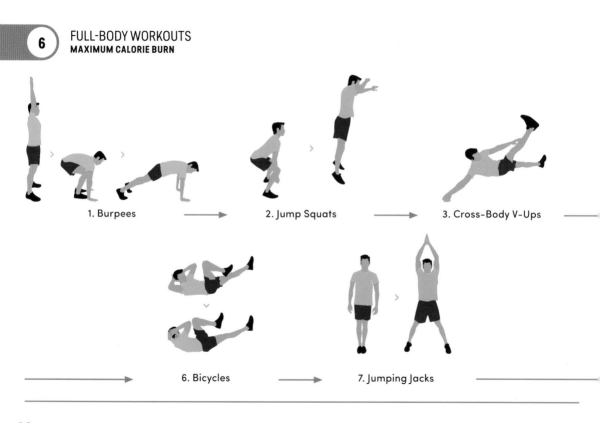

1. Burpees

2. Jump Squats

3. Cross-Body V-Ups

6. Bicycles

7. Jumping Jacks

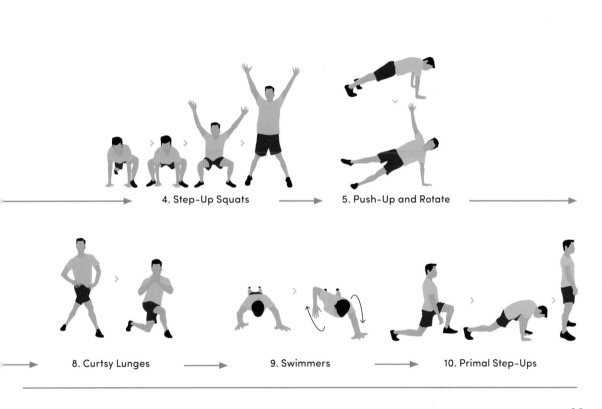

4. Step-Up Squats

5. Push-Up and Rotate

8. Curtsy Lunges

9. Swimmers

10. Primal Step-Ups

FULL-BODY WORKOUTS
MAXIMUM CALORIE BURN

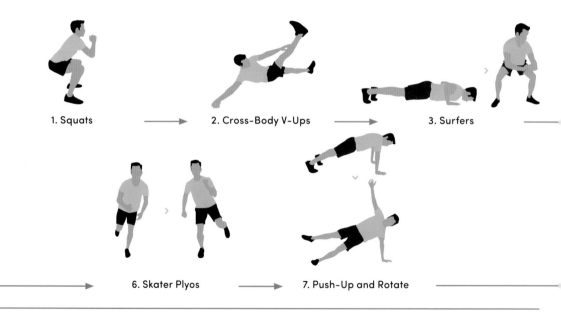

1. Squats

2. Cross-Body V-Ups

3. Surfers

6. Skater Plyos

7. Push-Up and Rotate

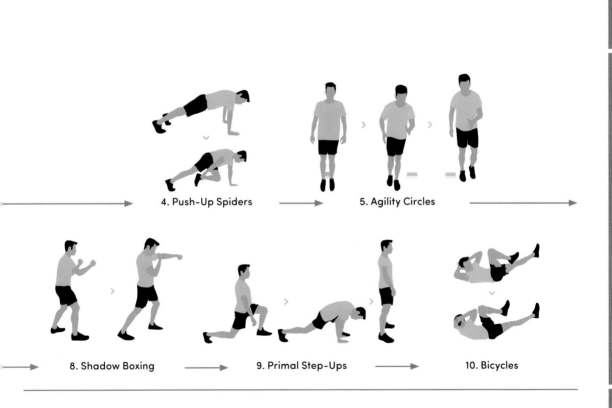

4. Push-Up Spiders

5. Agility Circles

8. Shadow Boxing

9. Primal Step-Ups

10. Bicycles

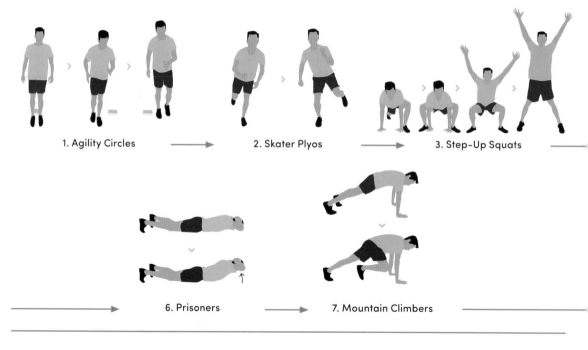

1. Agility Circles

2. Skater Plyos

3. Step-Up Squats

6. Prisoners

7. Mountain Climbers

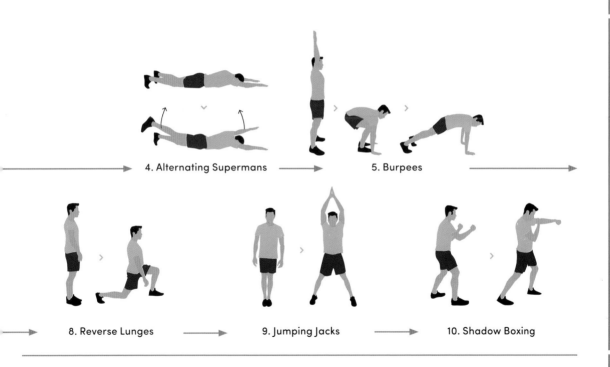

4. Alternating Supermans

5. Burpees

8. Reverse Lunges

9. Jumping Jacks

10. Shadow Boxing

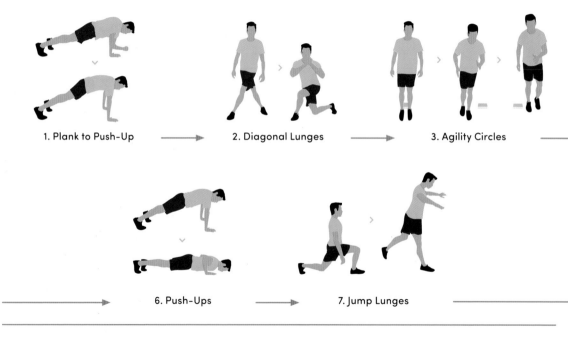

1. Plank to Push-Up ⟶ 2. Diagonal Lunges ⟶ 3. Agility Circles ⟶

⟶ 6. Push-Ups ⟶ 7. Jump Lunges ⟶

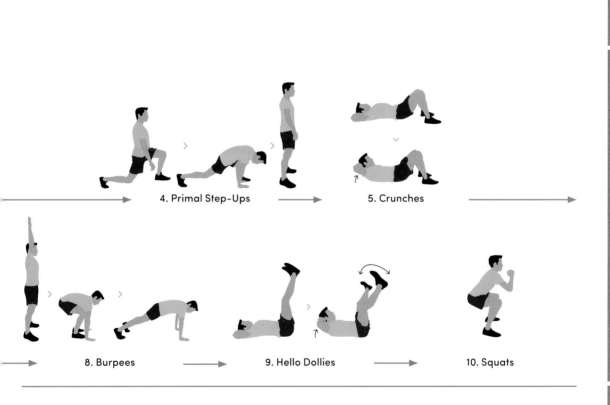

4. Primal Step-Ups

5. Crunches

8. Burpees

9. Hello Dollies

10. Squats

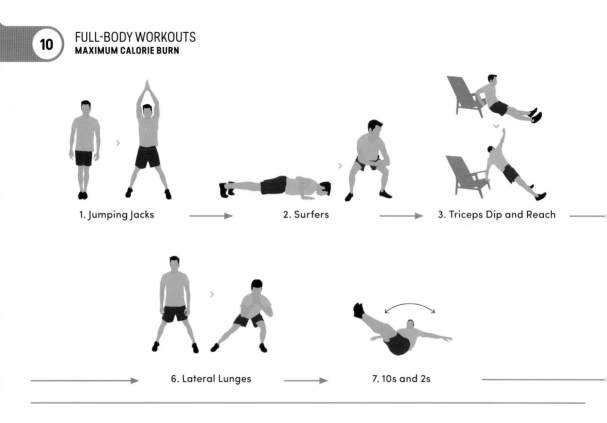

1. Jumping Jacks

2. Surfers

3. Triceps Dip and Reach

6. Lateral Lunges

7. 10s and 2s

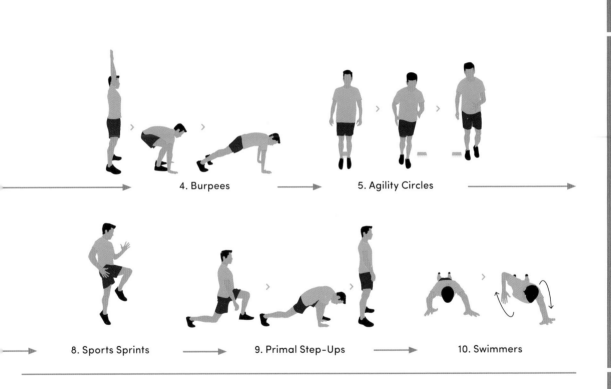

4. Burpees

5. Agility Circles

8. Sports Sprints

9. Primal Step-Ups

10. Swimmers

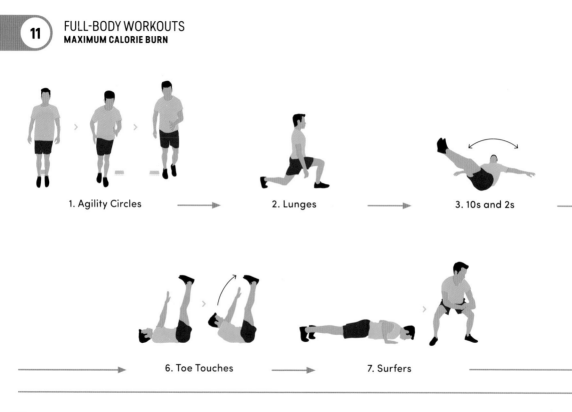

1. Agility Circles ➡️   2. Lunges ➡️   3. 10s and 2s

6. Toe Touches ➡️   7. Surfers

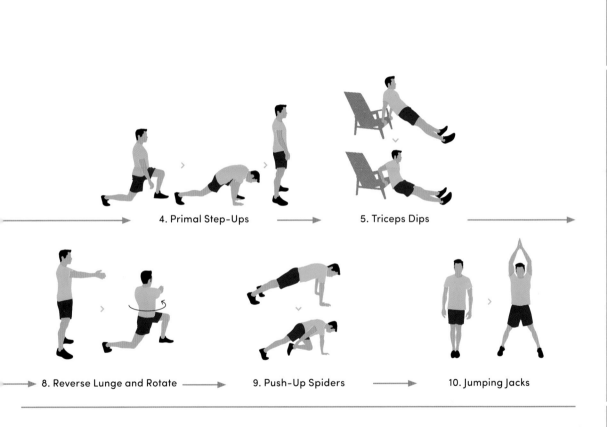

4. Primal Step-Ups

5. Triceps Dips

8. Reverse Lunge and Rotate

9. Push-Up Spiders

10. Jumping Jacks

FULL-BODY WORKOUTS
MAXIMUM CALORIE BURN

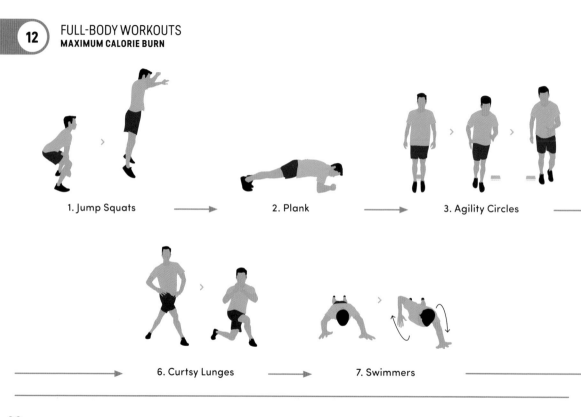

1. Jump Squats

2. Plank

3. Agility Circles

6. Curtsy Lunges

7. Swimmers

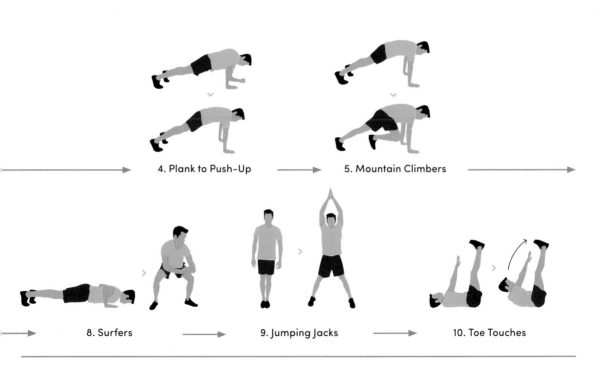

4. Plank to Push-Up

5. Mountain Climbers

8. Surfers

9. Jumping Jacks

10. Toe Touches

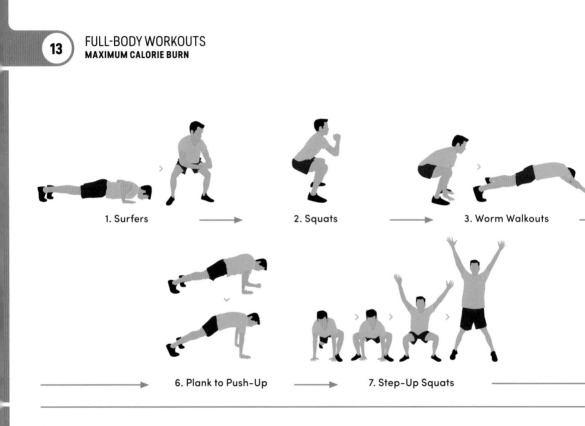

1. Surfers

2. Squats

3. Worm Walkouts

6. Plank to Push-Up

7. Step-Up Squats

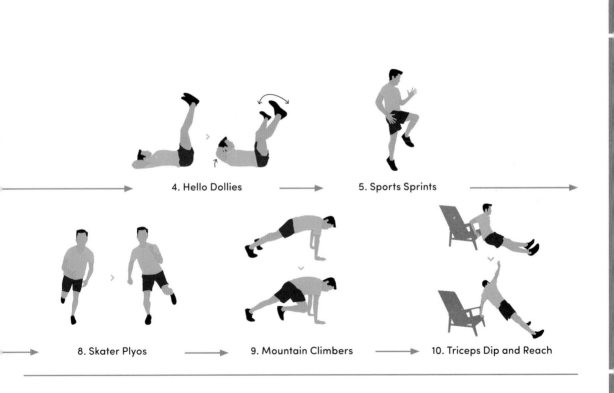

4. Hello Dollies

5. Sports Sprints

8. Skater Plyos

9. Mountain Climbers

10. Triceps Dip and Reach

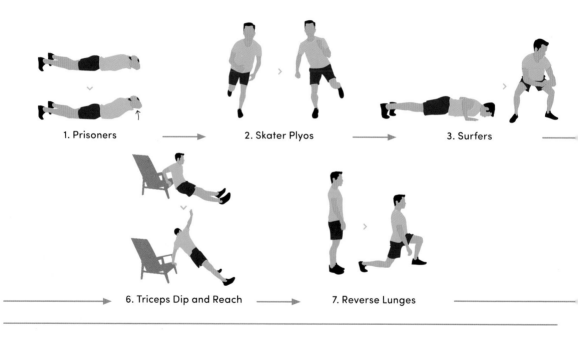

1. Prisoners

2. Skater Plyos

3. Surfers

6. Triceps Dip and Reach

7. Reverse Lunges

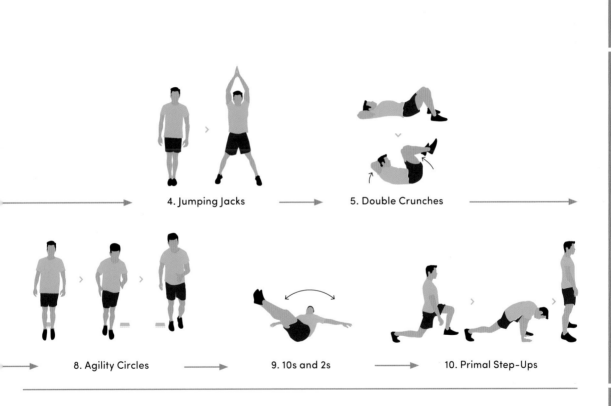

4. Jumping Jacks

5. Double Crunches

8. Agility Circles

9. 10s and 2s

10. Primal Step-Ups

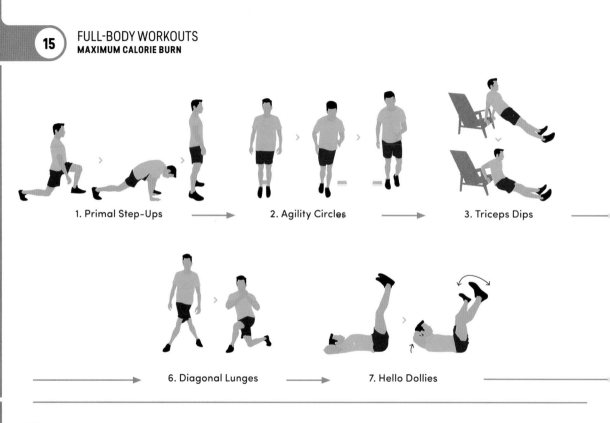

1. Primal Step-Ups

2. Agility Circles

3. Triceps Dips

6. Diagonal Lunges

7. Hello Dollies

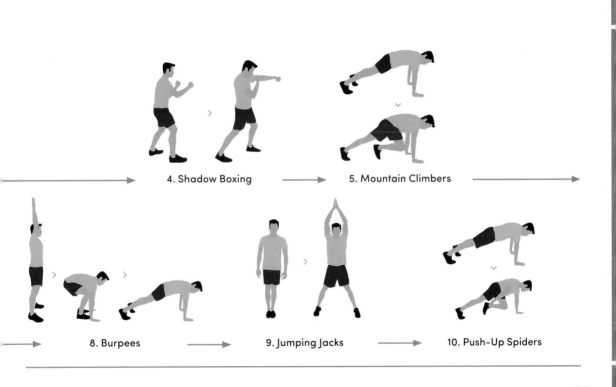

4. Shadow Boxing

5. Mountain Climbers

8. Burpees

9. Jumping Jacks

10. Push-Up Spiders

FULL-BODY WORKOUTS
MAXIMUM CALORIE BURN

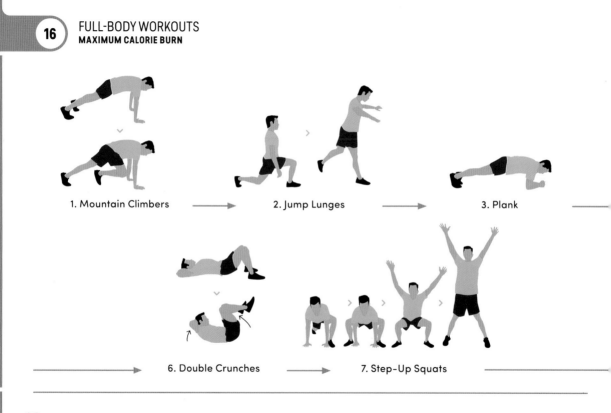

1. Mountain Climbers   ⟶   2. Jump Lunges   ⟶   3. Plank

6. Double Crunches   ⟶   7. Step-Up Squats

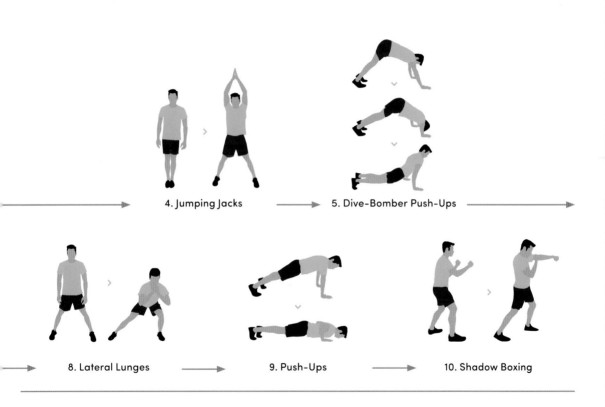

4. Jumping Jacks

5. Dive-Bomber Push-Ups

8. Lateral Lunges

9. Push-Ups

10. Shadow Boxing

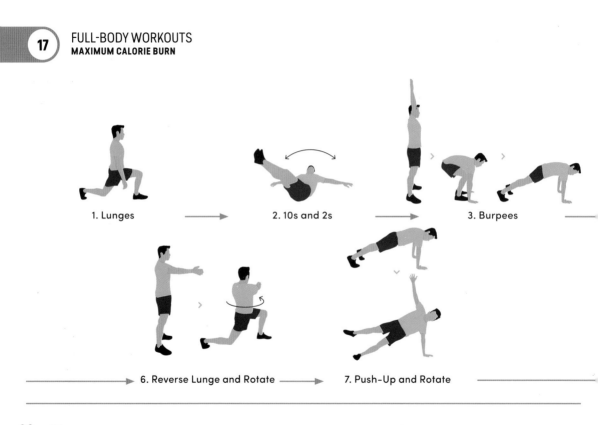

1. Lunges 2. 10s and 2s 3. Burpees

6. Reverse Lunge and Rotate 7. Push-Up and Rotate

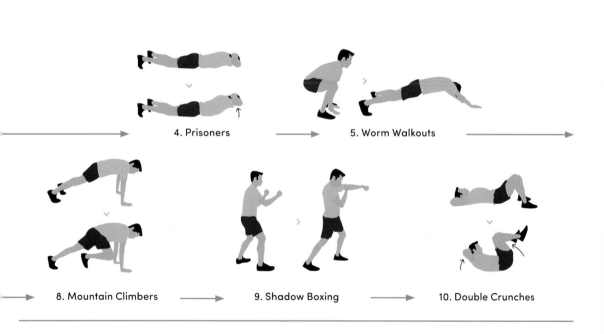

4. Prisoners

5. Worm Walkouts

8. Mountain Climbers

9. Shadow Boxing

10. Double Crunches

FULL-BODY WORKOUTS
MAXIMUM CALORIE BURN

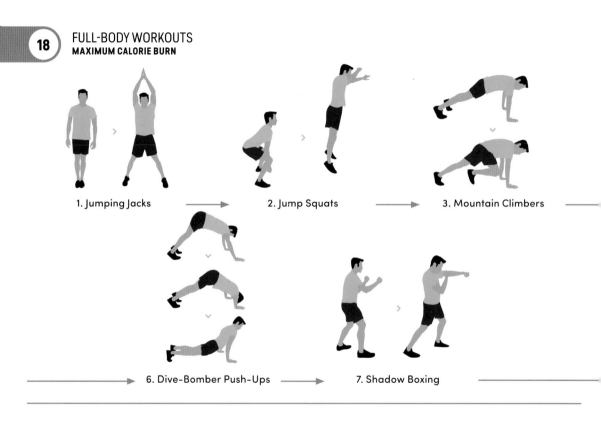

1. Jumping Jacks → 2. Jump Squats → 3. Mountain Climbers →

6. Dive-Bomber Push-Ups → 7. Shadow Boxing →

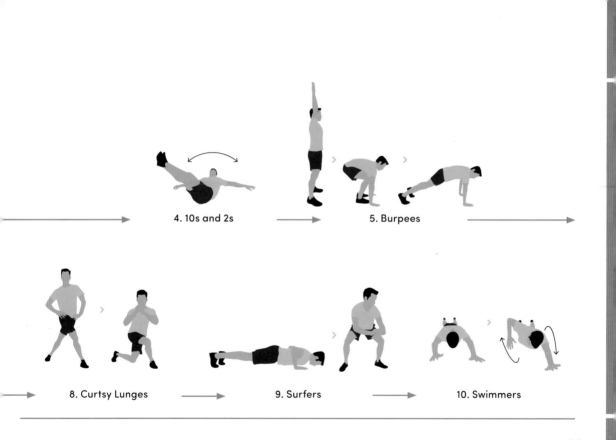

4. 10s and 2s

5. Burpees

8. Curtsy Lunges

9. Surfers

10. Swimmers

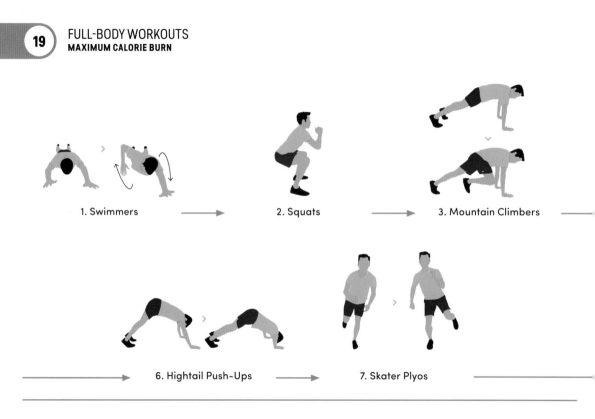

1. Swimmers

2. Squats

3. Mountain Climbers

6. Hightail Push-Ups

7. Skater Plyos

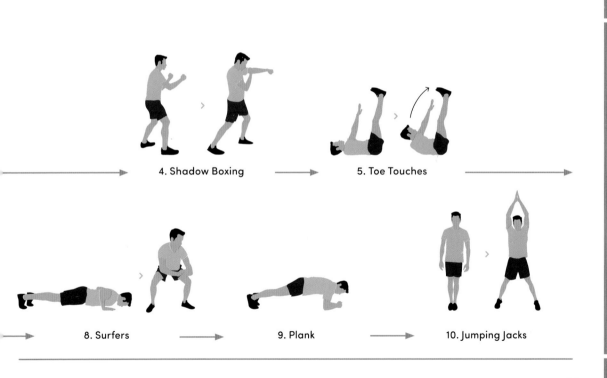

4. Shadow Boxing

5. Toe Touches

8. Surfers

9. Plank

10. Jumping Jacks

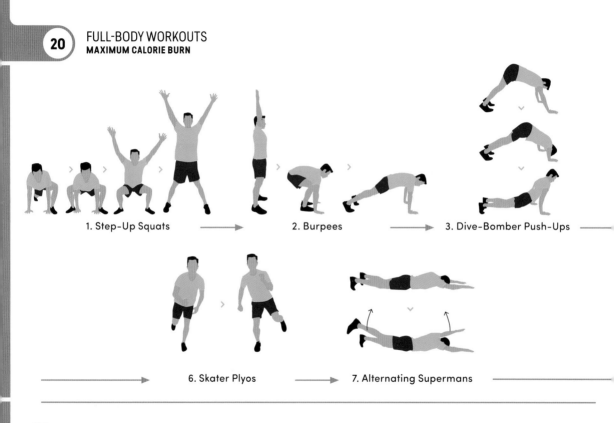

1. Step-Up Squats

2. Burpees

3. Dive-Bomber Push-Ups

6. Skater Plyos

7. Alternating Supermans

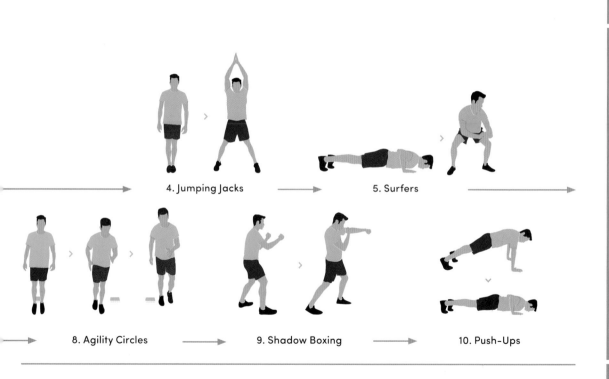

4. Jumping Jacks

5. Surfers

8. Agility Circles

9. Shadow Boxing

10. Push-Ups

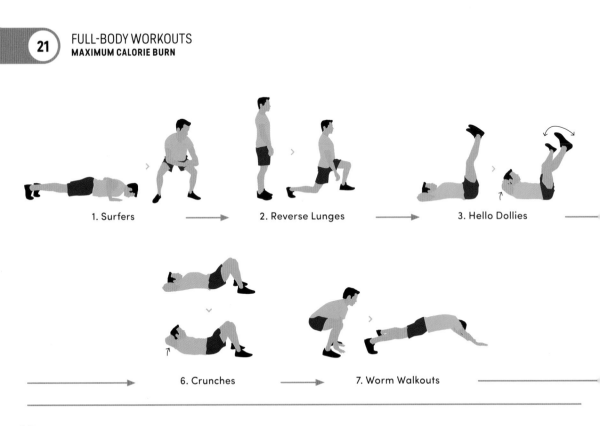

1. Surfers

2. Reverse Lunges

3. Hello Dollies

6. Crunches

7. Worm Walkouts

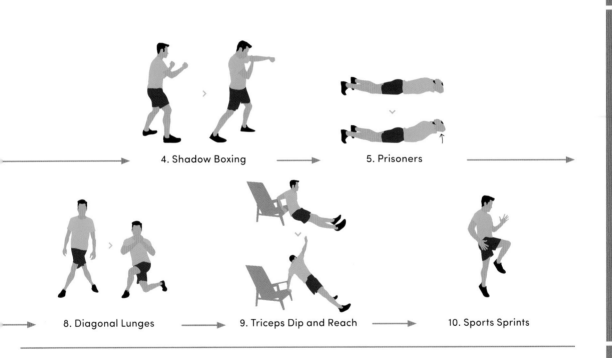

4. Shadow Boxing

5. Prisoners

8. Diagonal Lunges

9. Triceps Dip and Reach

10. Sports Sprints

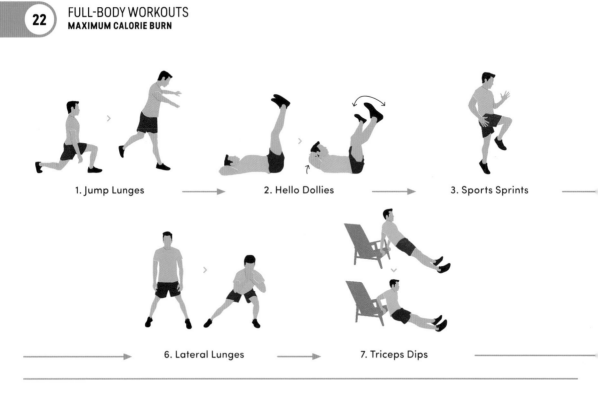

1. Jump Lunges

2. Hello Dollies

3. Sports Sprints

6. Lateral Lunges

7. Triceps Dips

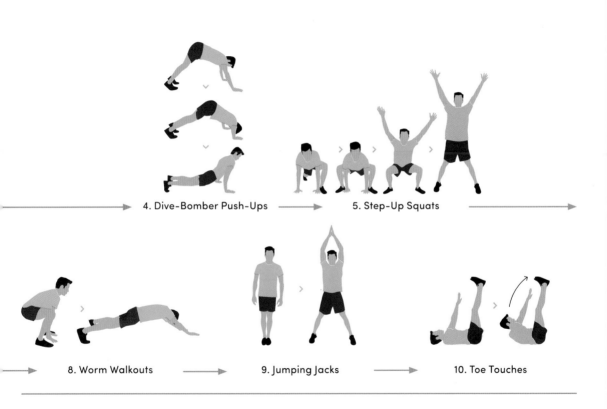

4. Dive-Bomber Push-Ups

5. Step-Up Squats

8. Worm Walkouts

9. Jumping Jacks

10. Toe Touches

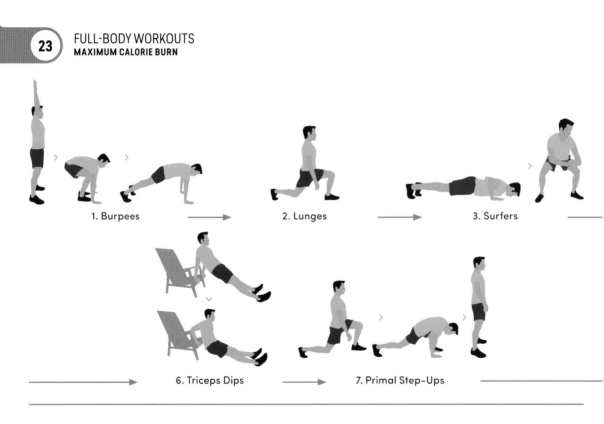

1. Burpees
2. Lunges
3. Surfers

6. Triceps Dips
7. Primal Step-Ups

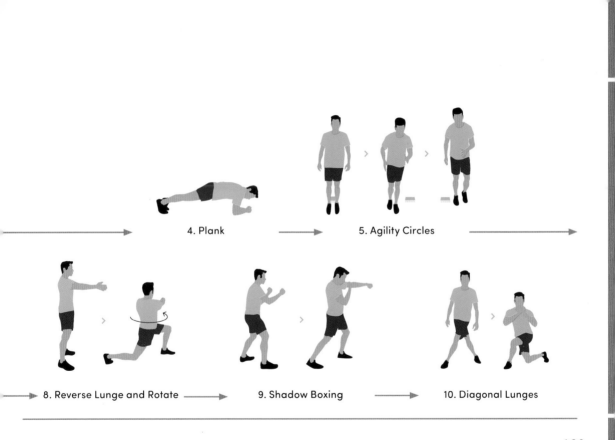

4. Plank

5. Agility Circles

8. Reverse Lunge and Rotate

9. Shadow Boxing

10. Diagonal Lunges

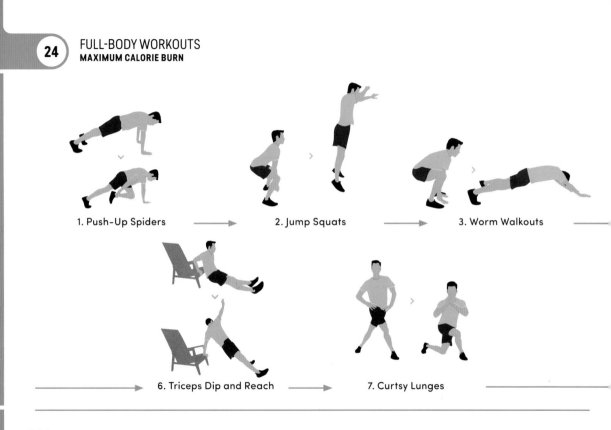

1. Push-Up Spiders

2. Jump Squats

3. Worm Walkouts

6. Triceps Dip and Reach

7. Curtsy Lunges

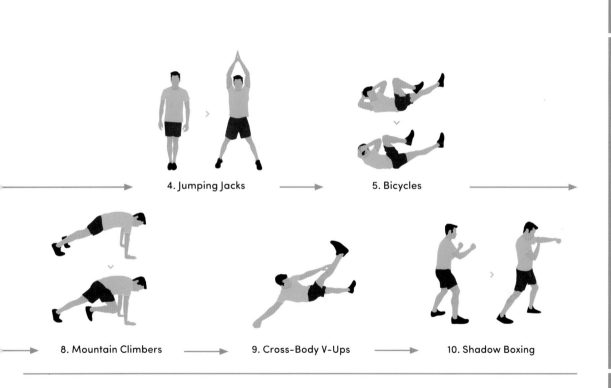

4. Jumping Jacks

5. Bicycles

8. Mountain Climbers

9. Cross-Body V-Ups

10. Shadow Boxing

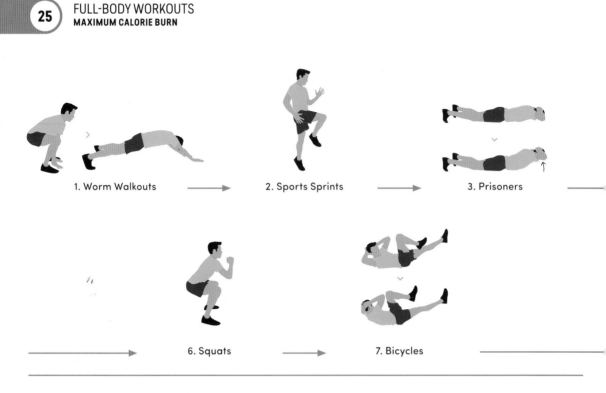

1. Worm Walkouts ⟶ 2. Sports Sprints ⟶ 3. Prisoners ⟶

⟶ 6. Squats ⟶ 7. Bicycles ⟶

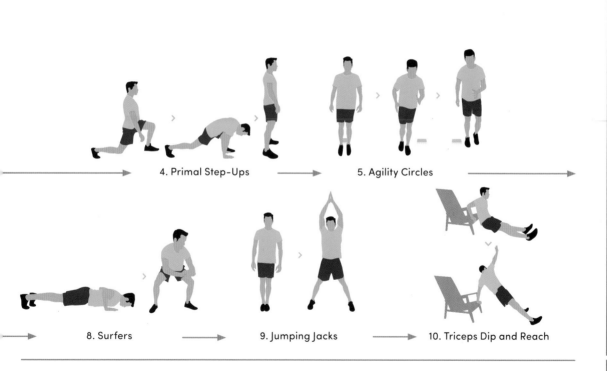

4. Primal Step-Ups

5. Agility Circles

8. Surfers

9. Jumping Jacks

10. Triceps Dip and Reach

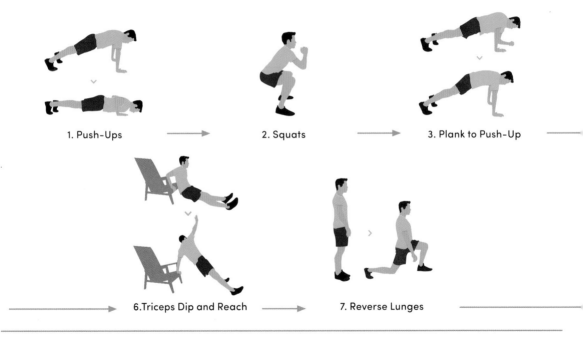

1. Push-Ups

2. Squats

3. Plank to Push-Up

6. Triceps Dip and Reach

7. Reverse Lunges

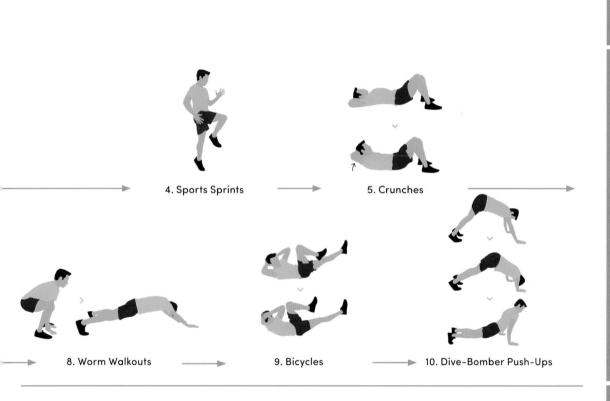

4. Sports Sprints

5. Crunches

8. Worm Walkouts

9. Bicycles

10. Dive-Bomber Push-Ups

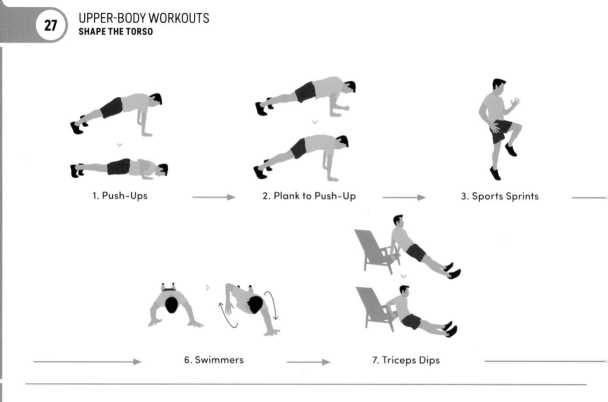

1. Push-Ups

2. Plank to Push-Up

3. Sports Sprints

6. Swimmers

7. Triceps Dips

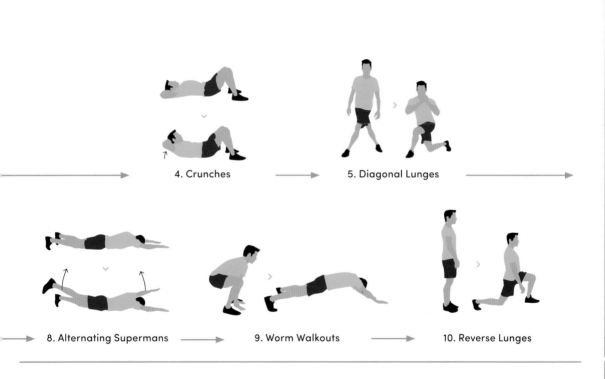

4. Crunches

5. Diagonal Lunges

8. Alternating Supermans

9. Worm Walkouts

10. Reverse Lunges

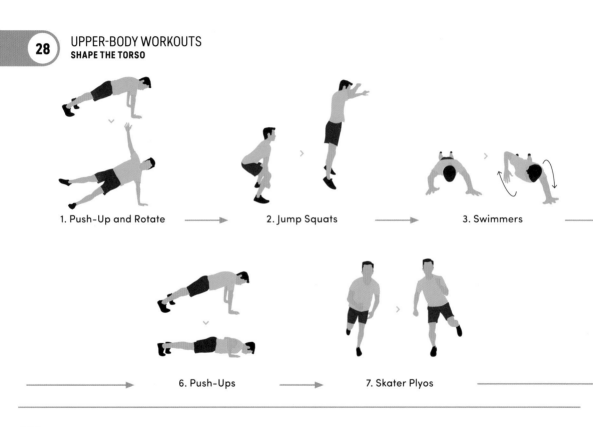

1. Push-Up and Rotate ⟶ 2. Jump Squats ⟶ 3. Swimmers ⟶

⟶ 6. Push-Ups ⟶ 7. Skater Plyos ⟶

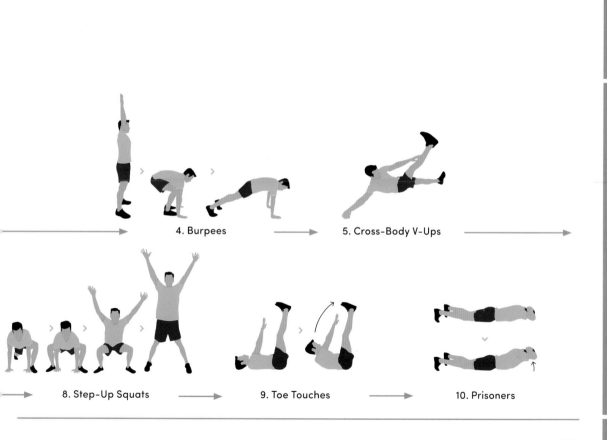

4. Burpees

5. Cross-Body V-Ups

8. Step-Up Squats

9. Toe Touches

10. Prisoners

UPPER-BODY WORKOUTS
SHAPE THE TORSO

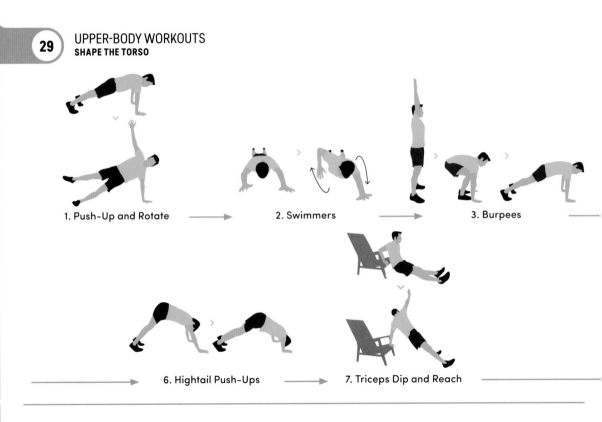

1. Push-Up and Rotate

2. Swimmers

3. Burpees

6. Hightail Push-Ups

7. Triceps Dip and Reach

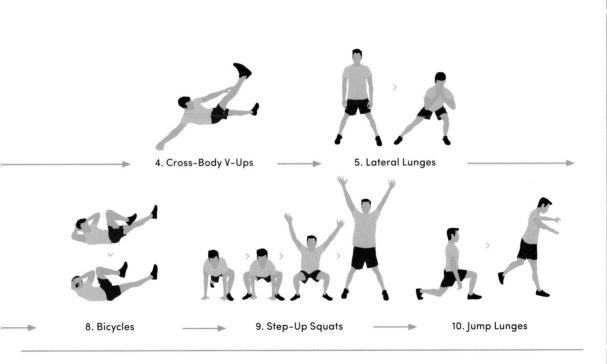

4. Cross-Body V-Ups

5. Lateral Lunges

8. Bicycles

9. Step-Up Squats

10. Jump Lunges

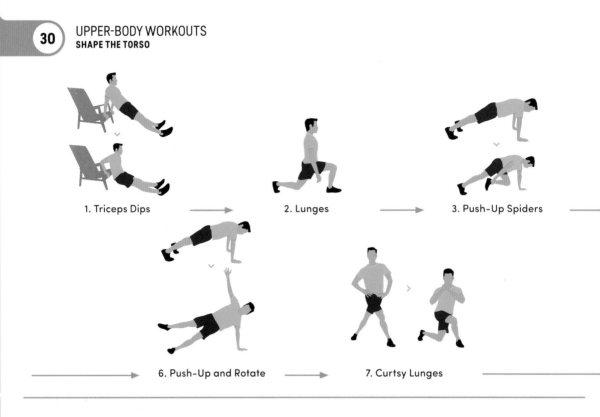

1. Triceps Dips   ⟶   2. Lunges   ⟶   3. Push-Up Spiders

6. Push-Up and Rotate   ⟶   7. Curtsy Lunges

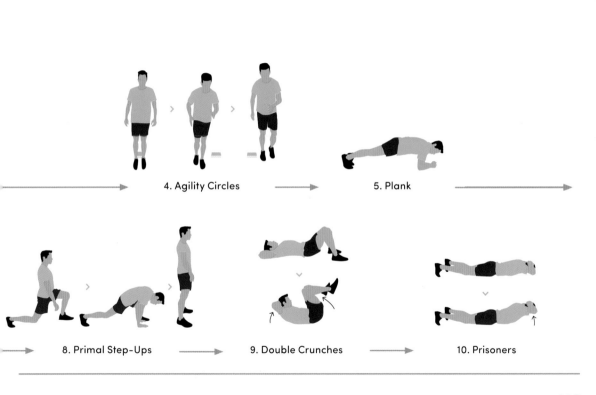

4. Agility Circles

5. Plank

8. Primal Step-Ups

9. Double Crunches

10. Prisoners

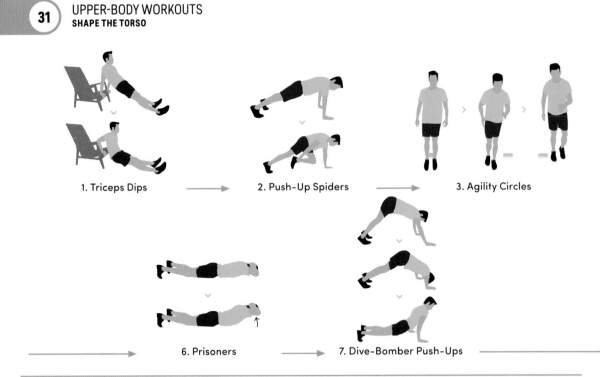

1. Triceps Dips

2. Push-Up Spiders

3. Agility Circles

6. Prisoners

7. Dive-Bomber Push-Ups

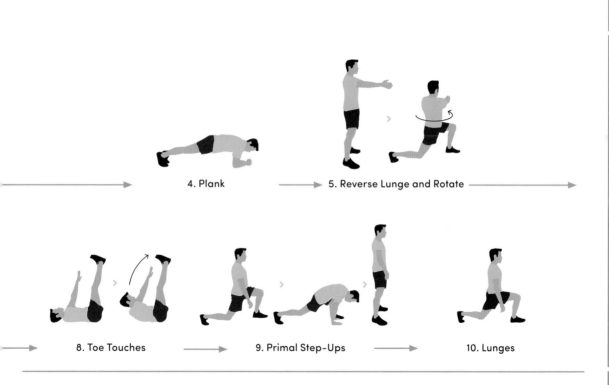

4. Plank

5. Reverse Lunge and Rotate

8. Toe Touches

9. Primal Step-Ups

10. Lunges

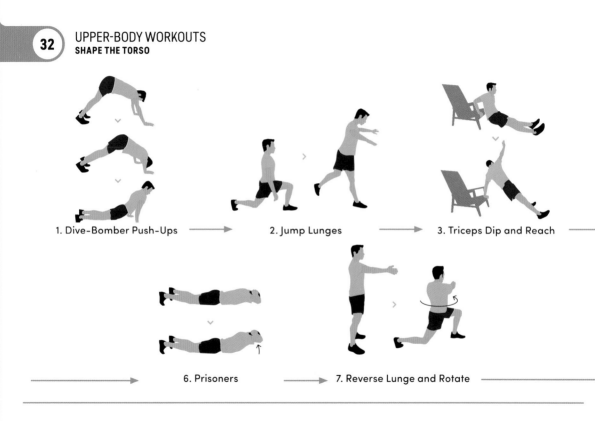

1. Dive-Bomber Push-Ups → 2. Jump Lunges → 3. Triceps Dip and Reach →

→ 6. Prisoners → 7. Reverse Lunge and Rotate →

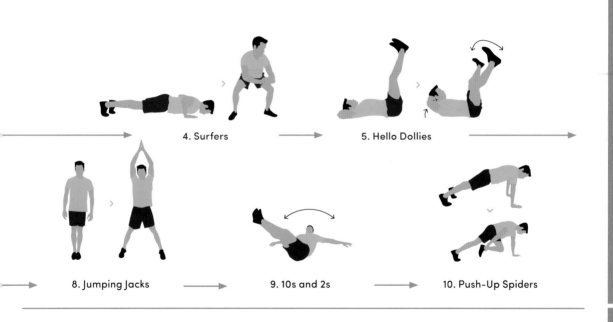

4. Surfers

5. Hello Dollies

8. Jumping Jacks

9. 10s and 2s

10. Push-Up Spiders

UPPER-BODY WORKOUTS
SHAPE THE TORSO

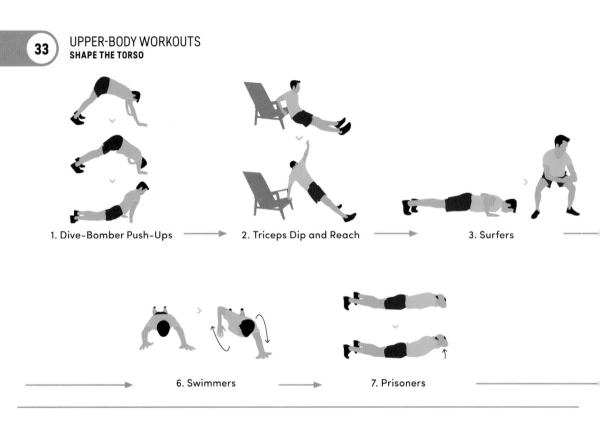

1. Dive-Bomber Push-Ups → 2. Triceps Dip and Reach → 3. Surfers →

→ 6. Swimmers → 7. Prisoners →

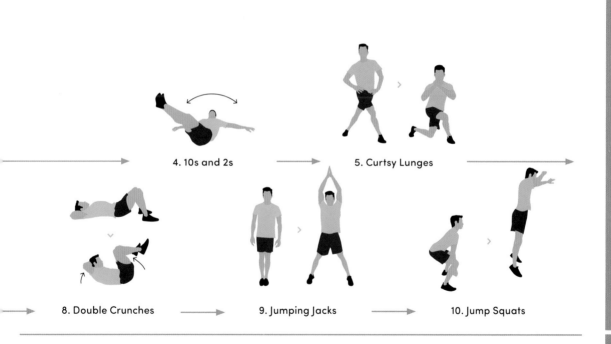

4. 10s and 2s

5. Curtsy Lunges

8. Double Crunches

9. Jumping Jacks

10. Jump Squats

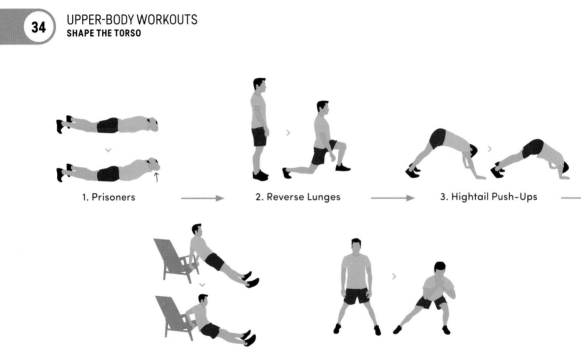

1. Prisoners

2. Reverse Lunges

3. Hightail Push-Ups

6. Triceps Dips

7. Lateral Lunges

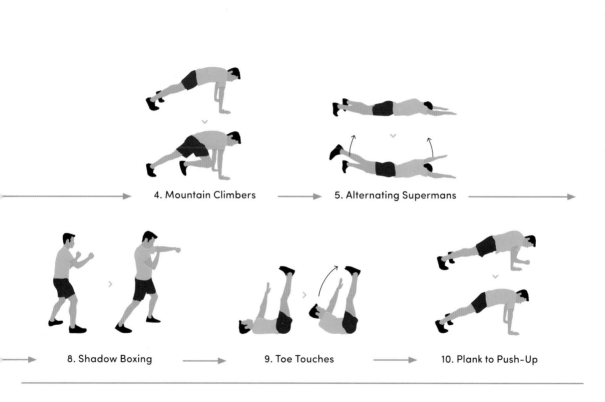

4. Mountain Climbers

5. Alternating Supermans

8. Shadow Boxing

9. Toe Touches

10. Plank to Push-Up

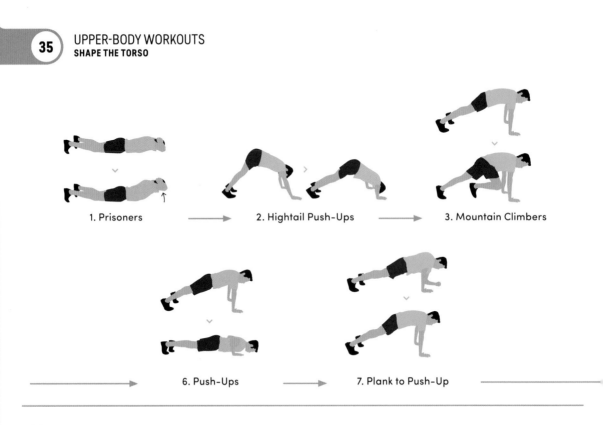

1. Prisoners → 2. Hightail Push-Ups → 3. Mountain Climbers

→ 6. Push-Ups → 7. Plank to Push-Up —

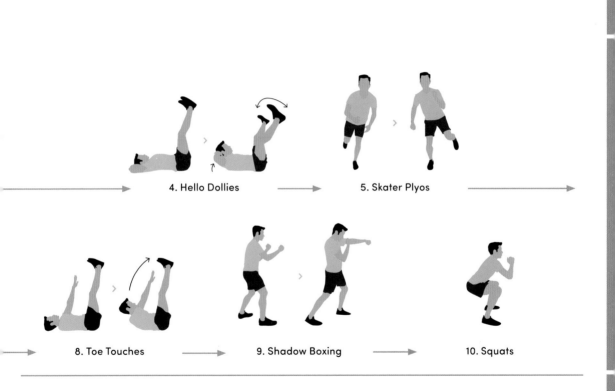

4. Hello Dollies

5. Skater Plyos

8. Toe Touches

9. Shadow Boxing

10. Squats

LOWER-BODY WORKOUTS
FLEXIBILITY AND TONE

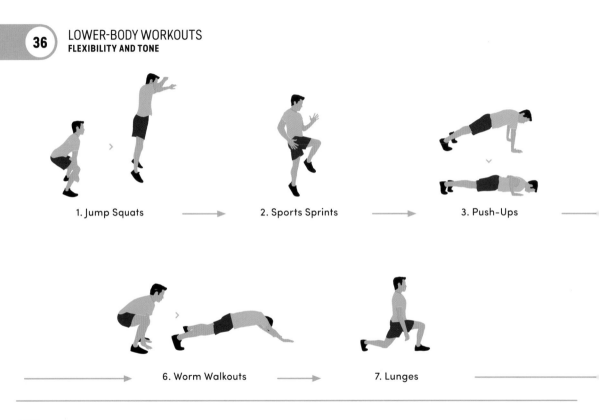

1. Jump Squats

2. Sports Sprints

3. Push-Ups

6. Worm Walkouts

7. Lunges

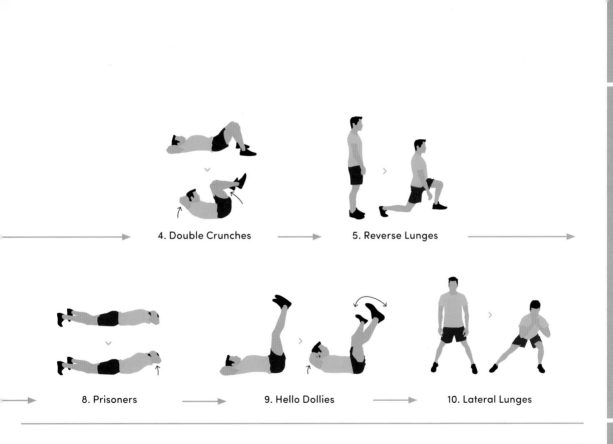

4. Double Crunches

5. Reverse Lunges

8. Prisoners

9. Hello Dollies

10. Lateral Lunges

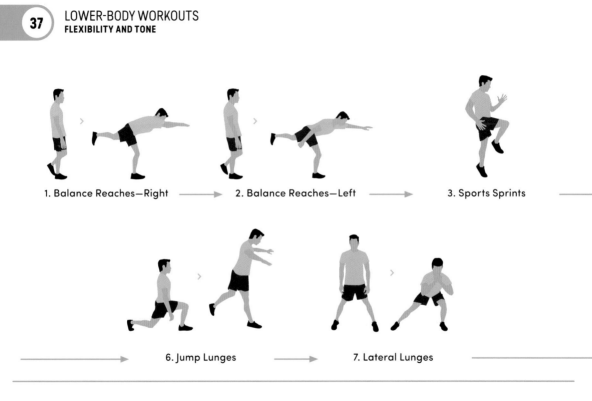

1. Balance Reaches—Right   2. Balance Reaches—Left   3. Sports Sprints

6. Jump Lunges   7. Lateral Lunges

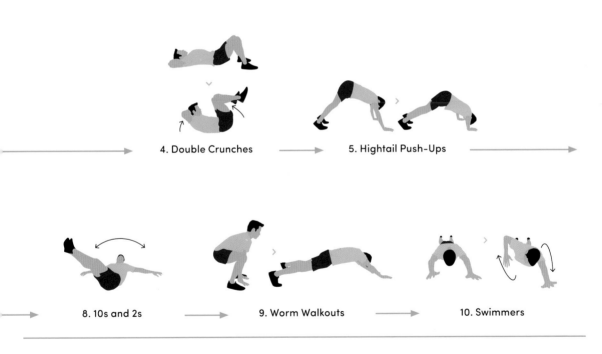

4. Double Crunches

5. Hightail Push-Ups

8. 10s and 2s

9. Worm Walkouts

10. Swimmers

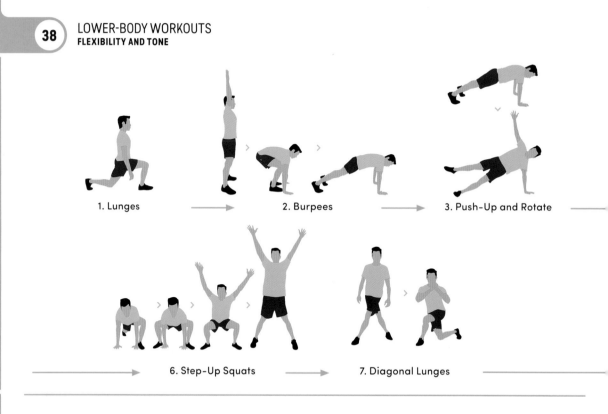

1. Lunges

2. Burpees

3. Push-Up and Rotate

6. Step-Up Squats

7. Diagonal Lunges

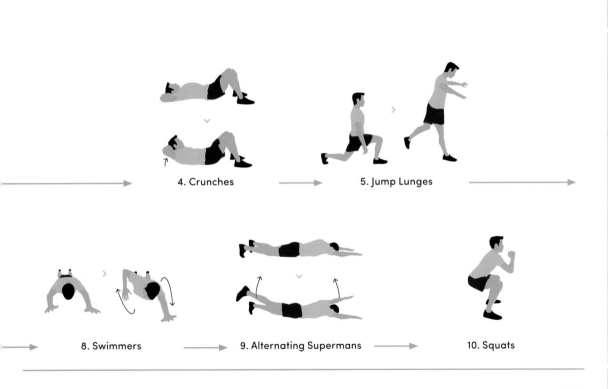

4. Crunches

5. Jump Lunges

8. Swimmers

9. Alternating Supermans

10. Squats

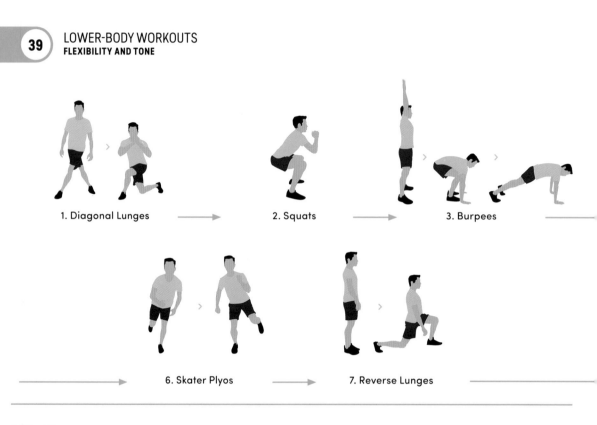

1. Diagonal Lunges

2. Squats

3. Burpees

6. Skater Plyos

7. Reverse Lunges

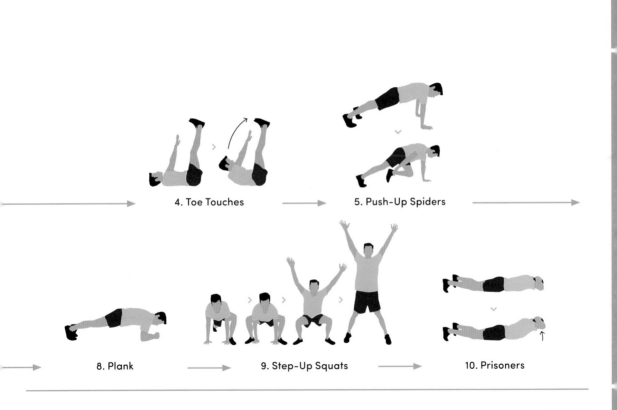

4. Toe Touches

5. Push-Up Spiders

8. Plank

9. Step-Up Squats

10. Prisoners

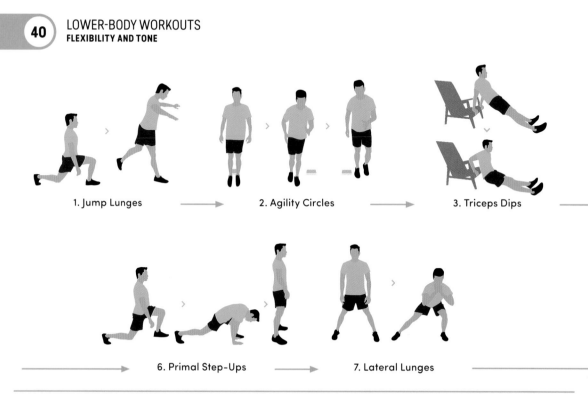

1. Jump Lunges

2. Agility Circles

3. Triceps Dips

6. Primal Step-Ups

7. Lateral Lunges

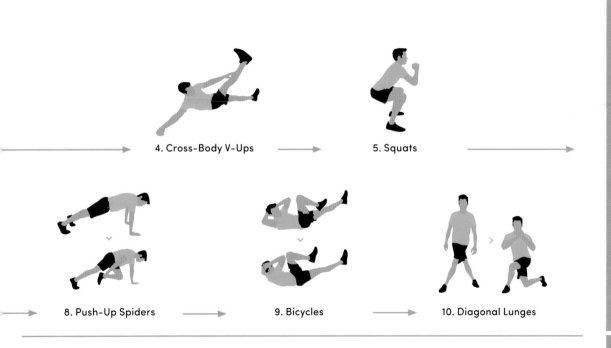

4. Cross-Body V-Ups

5. Squats

8. Push-Up Spiders

9. Bicycles

10. Diagonal Lunges

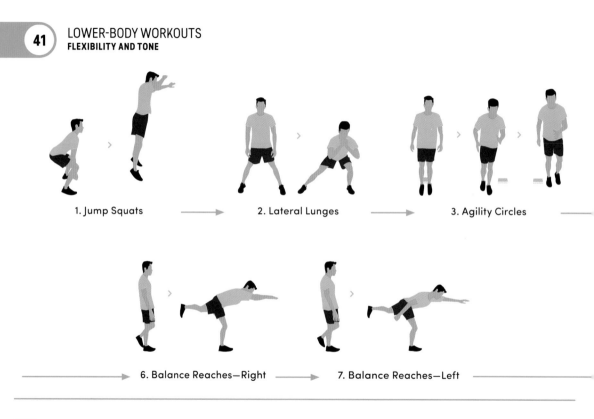

1. Jump Squats

2. Lateral Lunges

3. Agility Circles

6. Balance Reaches—Right

7. Balance Reaches—Left

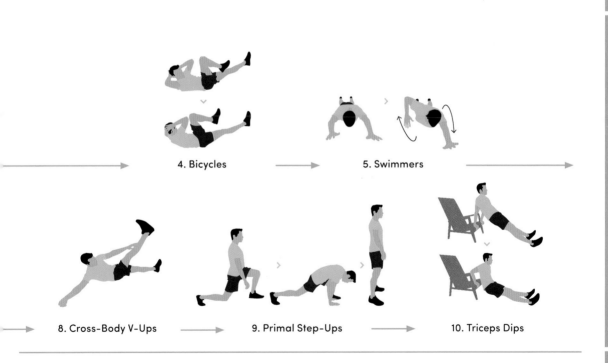

4. Bicycles

5. Swimmers

8. Cross-Body V-Ups

9. Primal Step-Ups

10. Triceps Dips

42

LOWER-BODY WORKOUTS
FLEXIBILITY AND TONE

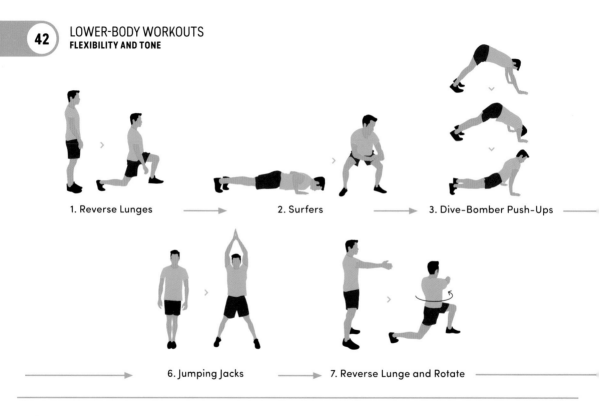

1. Reverse Lunges

2. Surfers

3. Dive-Bomber Push-Ups

6. Jumping Jacks

7. Reverse Lunge and Rotate

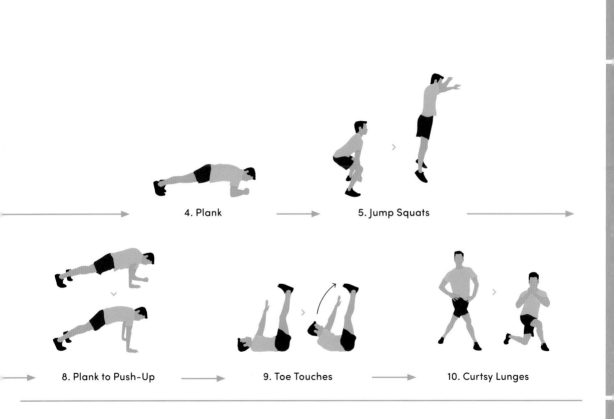

4. Plank

5. Jump Squats

8. Plank to Push-Up

9. Toe Touches

10. Curtsy Lunges

43

LOWER-BODY WORKOUTS
FLEXIBILITY AND TONE

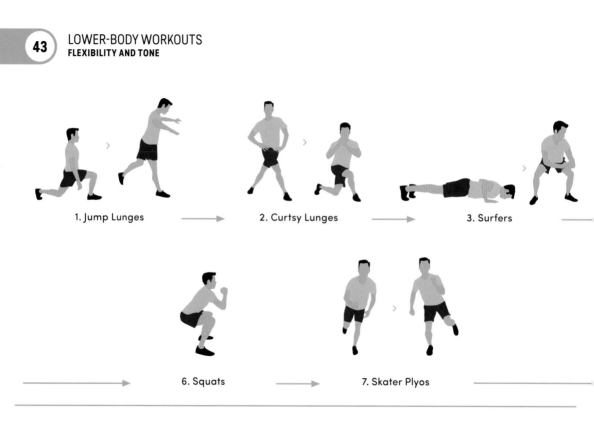

1. Jump Lunges   2. Curtsy Lunges   3. Surfers

6. Squats   7. Skater Plyos

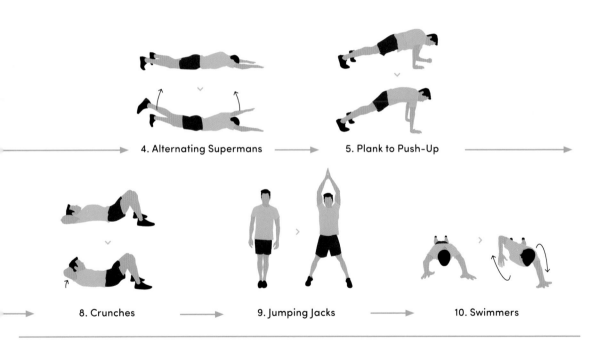

4. Alternating Supermans

5. Plank to Push-Up

8. Crunches

9. Jumping Jacks

10. Swimmers

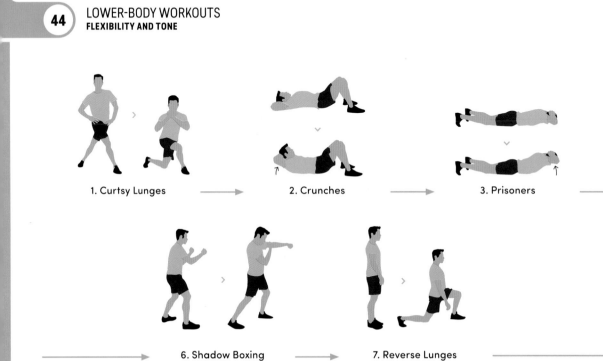

1. Curtsy Lunges

2. Crunches

3. Prisoners

6. Shadow Boxing

7. Reverse Lunges

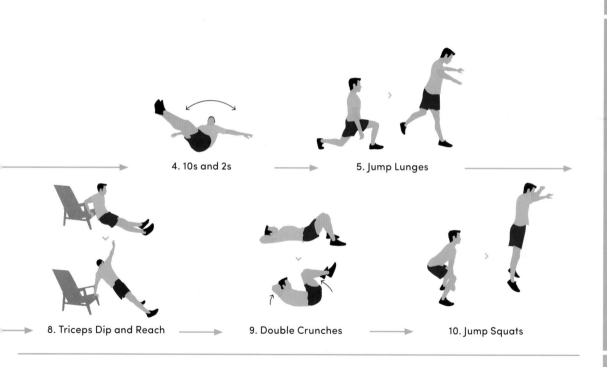

4. 10s and 2s

5. Jump Lunges

8. Triceps Dip and Reach

9. Double Crunches

10. Jump Squats

LOWER-BODY WORKOUTS
FLEXIBILITY AND TONE

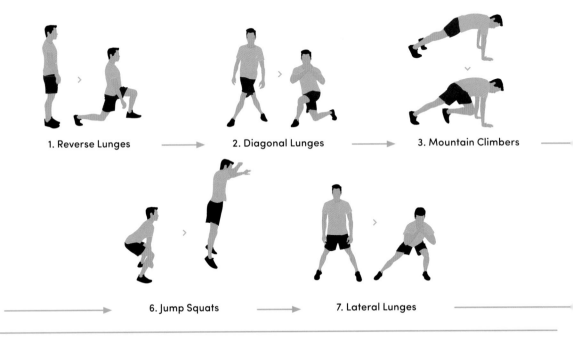

1. Reverse Lunges → 2. Diagonal Lunges → 3. Mountain Climbers →

6. Jump Squats → 7. Lateral Lunges →

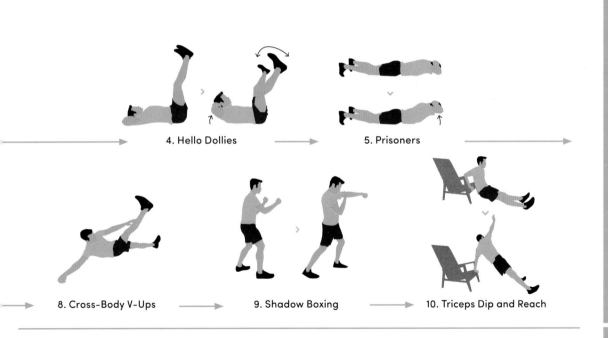

4. Hello Dollies

5. Prisoners

8. Cross-Body V-Ups

9. Shadow Boxing

10. Triceps Dip and Reach

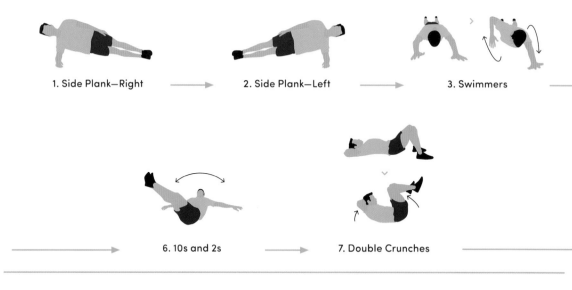

1. Side Plank—Right

2. Side Plank—Left

3. Swimmers

6. 10s and 2s

7. Double Crunches

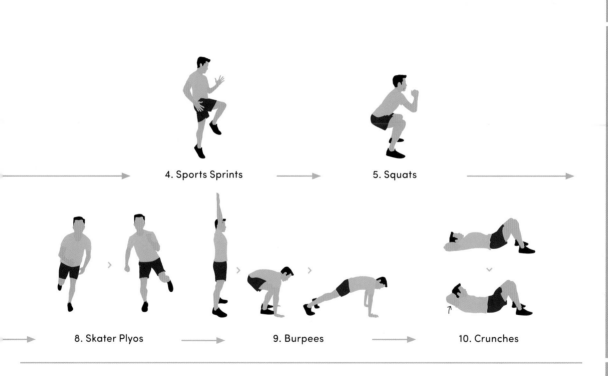

4. Sports Sprints

5. Squats

8. Skater Plyos

9. Burpees

10. Crunches

47

ABDOMINAL WORKOUTS
STRENGTHEN THE CORE

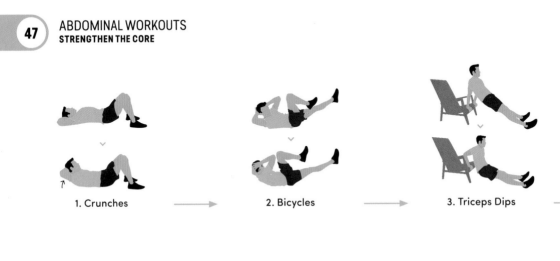

1. Crunches

2. Bicycles

3. Triceps Dips

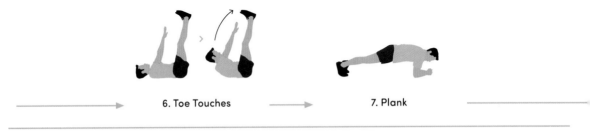

6. Toe Touches

7. Plank

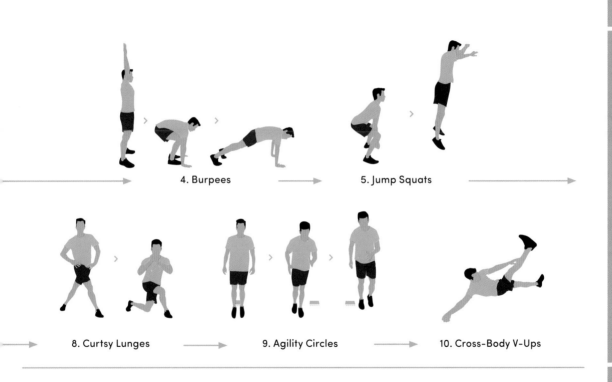

4. Burpees

5. Jump Squats

8. Curtsy Lunges

9. Agility Circles

10. Cross-Body V-Ups

48

ABDOMINAL WORKOUTS
STRENGTHEN THE CORE

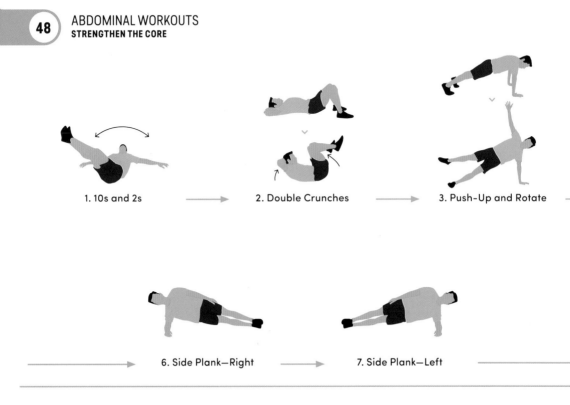

1. 10s and 2s

2. Double Crunches

3. Push-Up and Rotate

6. Side Plank—Right

7. Side Plank—Left

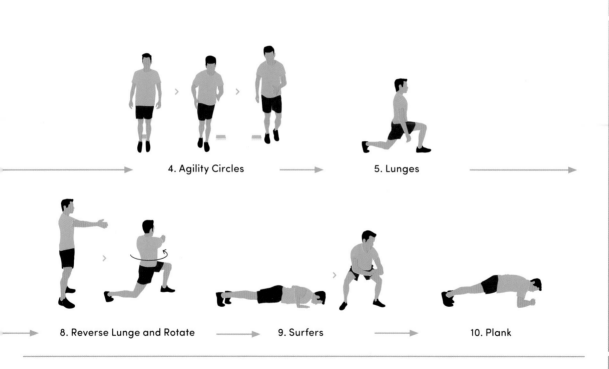

4. Agility Circles

5. Lunges

8. Reverse Lunge and Rotate

9. Surfers

10. Plank

49

ABDOMINAL WORKOUTS
STRENGTHEN THE CORE

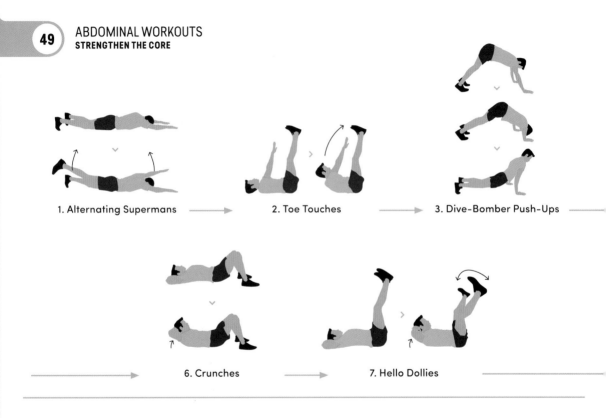

1. Alternating Supermans ⟶ 2. Toe Touches ⟶ 3. Dive-Bomber Push-Ups ⟶

⟶ 6. Crunches ⟶ 7. Hello Dollies ⟶

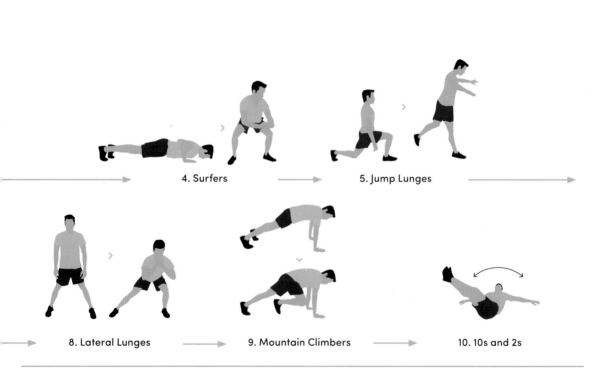

4. Surfers

5. Jump Lunges

8. Lateral Lunges

9. Mountain Climbers

10. 10s and 2s

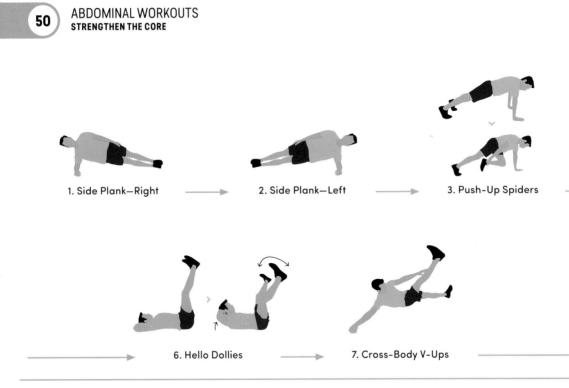

1. Side Plank—Right → 2. Side Plank—Left → 3. Push-Up Spiders

6. Hello Dollies → 7. Cross-Body V-Ups

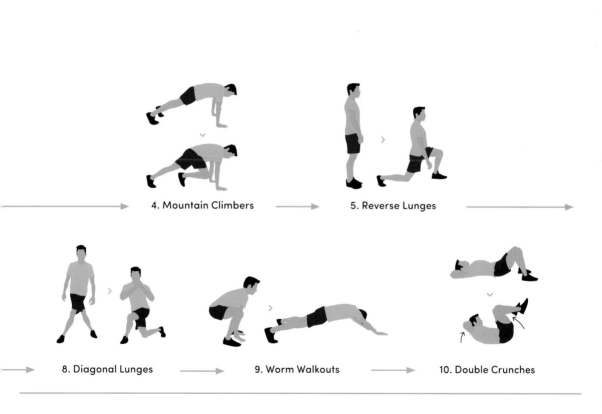

4. Mountain Climbers

5. Reverse Lunges

8. Diagonal Lunges

9. Worm Walkouts

10. Double Crunches

PART THREE

ADDING VARIATION TO YOUR PROGRAM

While the fifty workouts detailed in this book will keep your workout regime fresh for a long time, with a few adjustments you can continue to add challenges to these programs for months—even years! Here are some ways to modify the program to create new challenges, even after you've done all the workouts.

Time

Increase the work time for each movement to forty seconds. Do not change the rest time.

Repetitions	Weight vest or backpack	Supersets	Workout combinations
After you've increased the work time, try doing repetitions as slowly as possible. Try a "two seconds up, two seconds down" cadence. That would allow about ten repetitions in forty seconds. See if you can do it.	While bodyweight exercises are a convenient and highly effective way to get fit, you may reach a point of fitness where your own weight isn't challenging anymore. Instead of gaining weight (which is very rarely the goal of a program), add a weight vest or a backpack to increase the challenge of the exercises.	Instead of doing an exercise and resting ten seconds, do two or three exercises back to back with no rest. Absolutely none! One exercise flows into the next. After this is completed, rest for thirty seconds. This is a great challenge for advanced exercisers.	If you choose to do a circuit more than once (highly recommended for maximum results), do a different exercise circuit each time. For example, instead of completing circuit 1 three times, do circuit 1 once, circuit 2 once, and circuit 3 once. This gives you variety within your workout day.

Acknowledgments

I would like to thank my wife and soul mate, Lisa, and daughter, Madison, who bring a smile to my face every day; my parents, Linda and Larry, for raising me in a "culture of wellness"; my friends and colleagues in the fitness industry, especially Todd Durkin and my fitness family at Fitness Quest 10; my East Coast health and wellness family at The Human Performance Institute, who strive every day to improve human energy around the world; and all of those who have allowed me to be a part of their health and wellness journey.

Finally, to those who have disregarded their own health and fitness as a result of the overwhelming demands of daily life: this book is dedicated to offering an opportunity for time-strapped, busy adults to once again make health and wellness a part of their lives.